Hand and Upper Extremity Anatomy to Color and Study

Ray Poritsky, Ph.D. Emeritus
Department of Anatomy
Case Western Reserve University
Cleveland, Ohio

HANLEY & BELFUS, INC., Medical Publishers/Philadelphia

Publisher: HANLEY & BELFUS, INC.
Medical Publishers
210 South 13th Street
Philadelphia, PA 19107
215/546-7293, 800/962-1892
www.hanleyandbelfus.com

Library of Congress Cataloging-in-Publication Data

Hand and upper extremity anatomy to color and study/edited by Ray Poritsky.
   p. ; cm.
  ISBN 1-56053-372-2 (alk. paper)
  1. Arm—Anatomy—Atlases. 2. Hand—Anatomy—Atlases. 3. Coloring books. I.
Poritsky, Raphael.
  [DNLM: 1. Hand—anatomy & histology—Atlases. 2. Arm—anatomy &
histology—Atlases. WE 17 H236 2000]
  QM548 .H36 2000
  611'.97'0222—dc21
                                                                                                              99-052487

Hand and Upper Extremity Anatomy to Color and Study   ISBN 1-56053-372-2

© 2000 by Hanley & Belfus, Inc. All rights reserved. No part of this book may be reproduced, reused, republished, or transmitted in any form, or stored in a database or retrieval system, without written permission of the publisher.

Last digit is the print number: 9 8 7 6 5 4 3 2 1

Contents

1. Bones of the upper extremity, anterior aspect
2. Bones of the upper extremity, posterior aspect
3. Right scapula (shoulder blade)

Coracoid process and acromion (etymological cartoon)

4. The humerus
5. The radius and ulna
6. Bones of the hand (manus), palmar aspect, right hand
7. Bones of the hand (manus), dorsal aspect, right hand
8. Muscles of upper extremity I
9. Muscles of upper extremity II
10. Muscles of upper extremity III
11. Dissection of posterior shoulder and arm
12. Nerves and arteries of the posterior shoulder
13. Quadrangular space
14. Brachial plexus I: general plan
15. Brachial plexus and its nerves II
16. Arteries of the posterior shoulder and arm
17. Subclavian, axillary, and brachial arteries
18. Superficial veins and nerves of the anterior arm
19. Superficial veins and nerves of the posterior arm
20. Deep dissection of the posterior arm
21. Brachial plexus III
22. Nerves of the upper right limb, anterior aspect
23. Dissection of upper arm, anterior aspect
24. Biceps brachii: a flexor and supinator
25. Anterior forearm dissection
26. Arteries and nerves of the anterior forearm
27. Brachial plexus and major nerves of the arm
28. Pronator teres and superficial wrist flexors
29. Musculocutaneous nerve and the muscles it supplies
30. Muscular distribution of the median nerve
31. Flexor digitorum superficialis muscle
32. Flexor pollicis longus, flexor digitorum profundus, and median nerve
33. Median nerve and deep dissection of the forearm
34. Motor distribution of the ulnar nerve
35. Motor distribution of the radial nerve I, superficial muscles
36. Motor distribution of radial nerve II, deep muscles
37. Bones of the hand, palmar (ventral) aspect of right hand

Phalanx (etymological cartoon)

38. Palmar aponeurosis and anchoring connective tissue
39. Flexor retinaculum and superficial hand muscles
40. Deep thenar, hypothenar, and interosseous muscles
41. Interosseous and related muscles
42. Arteries of the hand
43. Deep palmar arch and deep branch of ulnar nerve
44. Nerves and arteries of the palm
45. Superficial palmar arch: median and ulnar nerves
46. Extensor tendons on dorsum of hand I
47. Extensor tendons on dorsum of hand II
48. Radial artery and superficial branch of radial nerve
49. Dorsum of hand
50. Palmar hand: deep dissection
51. Synovial flexor tendon sheaths
52. Synovial extensor tendon sheaths
53. Thumb muscles I
54. Thumb muscles II
55. Palmar interosseous muscles
56. Dorsal interosseous muscles of the hand
57. Some finger movements
58. Cutaneous nerve distribution on front of arm
59. Distribution of cutaneous nerves on back of upper limb
60. Muscle attachments of the anterior arm
61. Muscle attachments of the posterior arm
62. Muscle attachments of the anterior hand
63. Frontal (coronal) section of the right wrist and hand
64. Coronal section of the right shoulder
65. Ligaments of right shoulder joint, anterior aspect
66. Ligaments of right shoulder joint, posterior aspect
67. Ligaments of right elbow, ulnar side
68. Ligaments of right elbow, anterior aspect
69. Sagittal section of right elbow, radial side
70. Frontal section of right elbow
71. Ligaments of right wrist, palmar aspect
72. Ligaments of right wrist, posterior aspect
73. Hand dissection, oblique view, palmar aspect
74. Wrist cross-section
75. Hand cross-section I
76. Hand cross-section II
77. Unlabelled bones of the hand for self study, ventral aspect
78. Unlabelled bones of the hand for self study, dorsal aspect

Preface

This book is designed to help students learn the complex anatomy of the upper extremity. It also serves as a comprehensive review for students at the completion of their gross anatomy course. The various muscles, nerves, and blood vessels of the upper limb are depicted in bold black and white drawings for the reader to label and color. The reader may wish to simply identify each structure by its name and not color it. The use of color, however, will help delineate the structure in question, such as a muscle, or in the case of a vessel or nerve, adding color will more clearly reveal its path and distribution. Indeed, labelling each structure and adding color calls upon the reader to play a more active role rather than simply reading about anatomy in a book. I hope that this book will make it easier to master the anatomy of the upper limb. I also welcome suggestions and comments from readers.

I have used many of the beautiful pen and ink drawings by Eycleshymer and Jones published in 1925 in their classic *Hand Atlas of Clinical Anatomy*. These clear concise drawings were an outgrowth of their very popular *Manual of Surgical Anatomy* prepared for the army and navy medical corps during the First World War. I have updated the Latin names and relabelled them with current anatomical terms. In most of their drawings, I have added new leaders (connecting lines). In a few cases, I have modified the Eycleshymer and Jones drawings to include present day anatomical knowledge.

I have included a few etymological cartoons that I hope will afford a little levity in what can be, at times, a challenging subject, the anatomy of the upper limb. The knowledge of how each part of the body got its name is actually quite interesting and often makes it easier to remember that particular anatomy.

Color pencils at the ready! Go and Good Luck!

RAY PORITSKY, PH.D.
Cleveland, Ohio

Acknowledgments

Additional figures were drawn by Cheryl Owens and Wayne Timmerman. Most of the illustrations are reworked and updated figures from Eycleshymer and Jones: *Hand Atlas of Clinical Anatomy*, Lea & Febiger, 1925. Atlases and texts that I used to draw figures for this book are: Wolf-Heidegger: *Atlas of Systemic Human Anatomy*, Hafner, 1962; Spalteholz and Spanner: *Atlas of Human Anatomy, 16th ed.*, F.A. Davis, 1961; Hollinshead and Rosse: *Textbook of Anatomy, 4th ed.*, Harper and Row, 1985; Clemente: *A Regional Atlas of the Human Body, 3rd ed.*, Urban & Schwarzenberg, 1987; Töndury, *Angewandte und Topographische Anatomie*, Fretz & Wasmuth, 1949; Williams (ed): *Gray's Anatomy, 38th British ed.*, Churchill Livingstone, 1995; Netter: *The Ciba Collection of Medical Illustrations*, Ciba Pharmaceutical Company, 1959.

I wish to thank my publisher and editor, Linda Belfus, for her generous support and encouragement for this book and to her most helpful staff at Hanley and Belfus in Philadelphia, especially Denise Roslonski.

I thank and warmly dedicate this book to my wife Connie.

1 Bones of the upper extremity

Anterior aspect

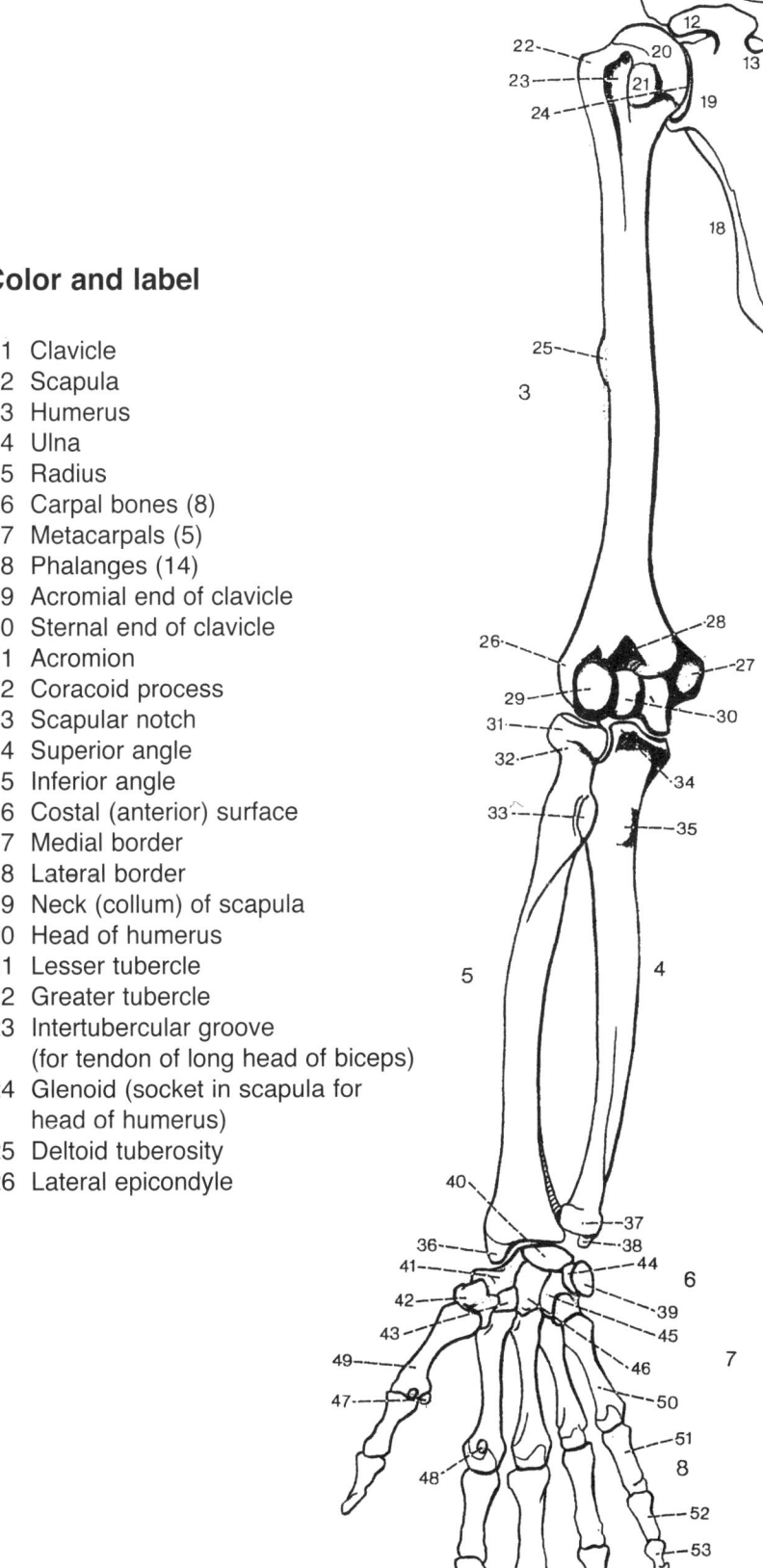

Color and label

1. Clavicle
2. Scapula
3. Humerus
4. Ulna
5. Radius
6. Carpal bones (8)
7. Metacarpals (5)
8. Phalanges (14)
9. Acromial end of clavicle
10. Sternal end of clavicle
11. Acromion
12. Coracoid process
13. Scapular notch
14. Superior angle
15. Inferior angle
16. Costal (anterior) surface
17. Medial border
18. Lateral border
19. Neck (collum) of scapula
20. Head of humerus
21. Lesser tubercle
22. Greater tubercle
23. Intertubercular groove (for tendon of long head of biceps)
24. Glenoid (socket in scapula for head of humerus)
25. Deltoid tuberosity
26. Lateral epicondyle
27. Medial epicondyle
28. Coronoid fossa
29. Capitulum of humerus
30. Trochlea of humerus
31. Head of radius
32. Neck of radius
33. Radial tuberosity (for insertion of biceps brachii)
34. Coronoid process of ulna
35. Tuberosity of ulna (for insertion of brachialis muscle)
36. Styloid process of radius
37. Head of ulna
38. Styloid process of ulna
39. Pisiform
40. Lunate
41. Scaphoid
42. Trapezium
43. Trapezoid
44. Triquetral
45. Hamate
46. Capitate
47. Sesamoid bones of thumb
48. Sesamoid bone of index finger
49. First metacarpal
50. Fifth metacarpal
51. Proximal phalanx of little finger (digiti minimi)
52. Middle phalanx
53. Terminal phalanx

2 Bones of the upper extremity

Posterior aspect

Color and label

1. Clavicle (collar bone)
2. Scapula (shoulder blade)
3. Humerus
4. Ulna
5. Radius
6. Medial border of scapula
7. Lateral border of scapula
8. Superior border of scapula
9. Superior angle of scapula
10. Inferior angle of scapula
11. Lateral angle (glenoid cavity)
12. Spine of scapula
13. Acromion
14. Scapular notch
15. Coracoid process
16. Supraspinous fossa (supraspinatus fossa)
17. Infraspinous fossa (infraspinatus fossa)
18. Infraglenoid tubercle
19. Neck of scapula
20. Head of humerus
21. Anatomical neck of humerus
22. Surgical neck of humerus (usual site of proximal humerus fracture)
23. Deltoid tuberosity
24. Medial epicondyle of humerus
25. Lateral epicondyle of humerus
26. Radial groove for radial nerve
27. Olecranon fossa
28. Sulcus for ulnar nerve
29. Olecranon of ulna
30. Head of radius
31. Neck of radius
32. Styloid process of ulna
33. Styloid process of radius
34. Pisiform (carpal) bone
35. Triquetral (carpal) bone
36. Lunate bone (most frequently dislocated wrist bone)
37. Scaphoid bone (most frequently fractured wrist bone)
38. Hamate (carpal) bone
39. Capitate (carpal) bone
40. Trapezoid (carpal) bone
41. Trapezium (carpal) bone
42. Metacarpal bones
43. Proximal phalanges
44. Middle phalanges
45. Distal phalanges

* Most frequent site of fracture of the clavicle (which is the most frequently broken bone)

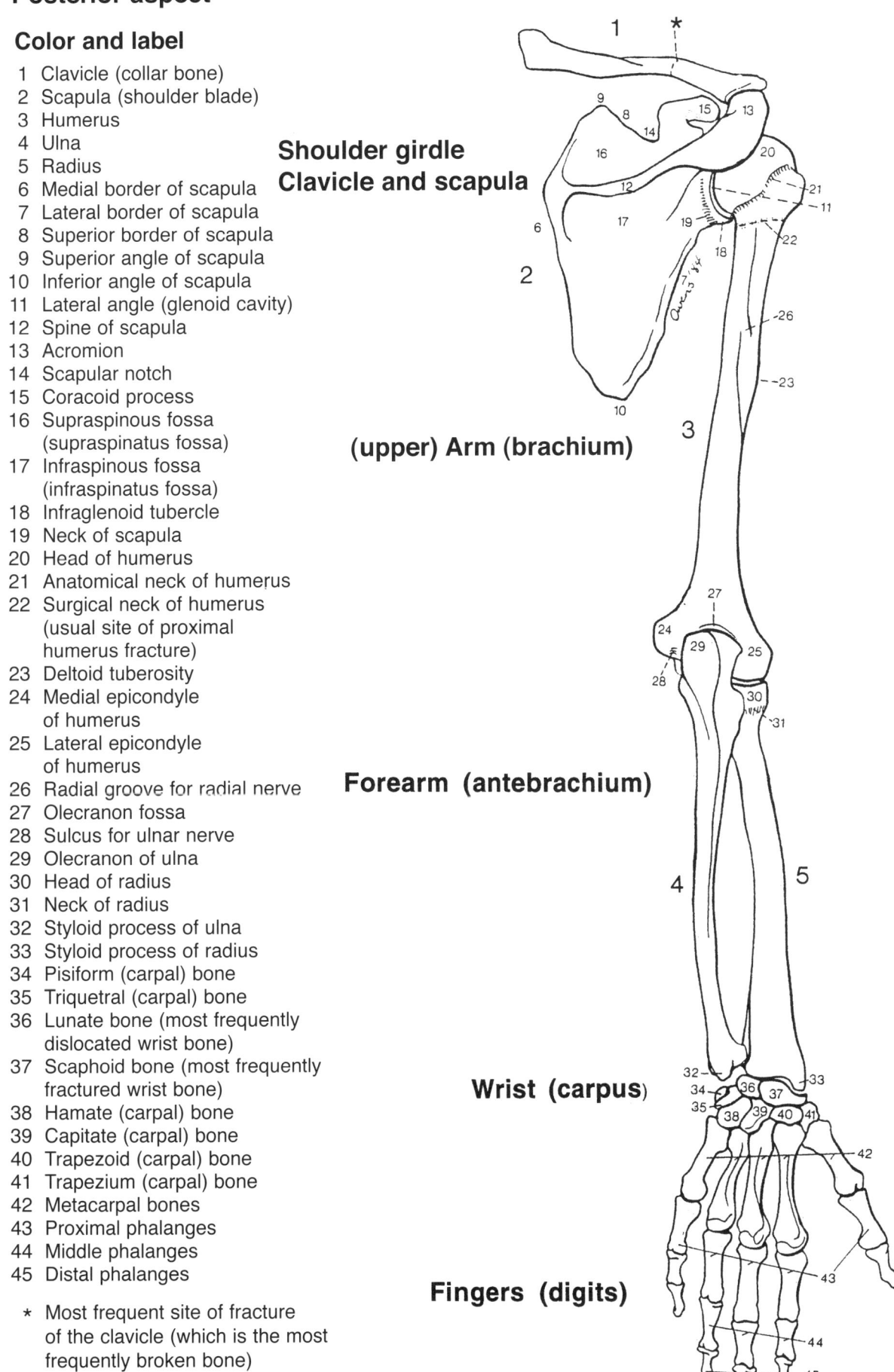

Shoulder girdle
Clavicle and scapula

(upper) Arm (brachium)

Forearm (antebrachium)

Wrist (carpus)

Fingers (digits)

3 Right scapula (shoulder blade)

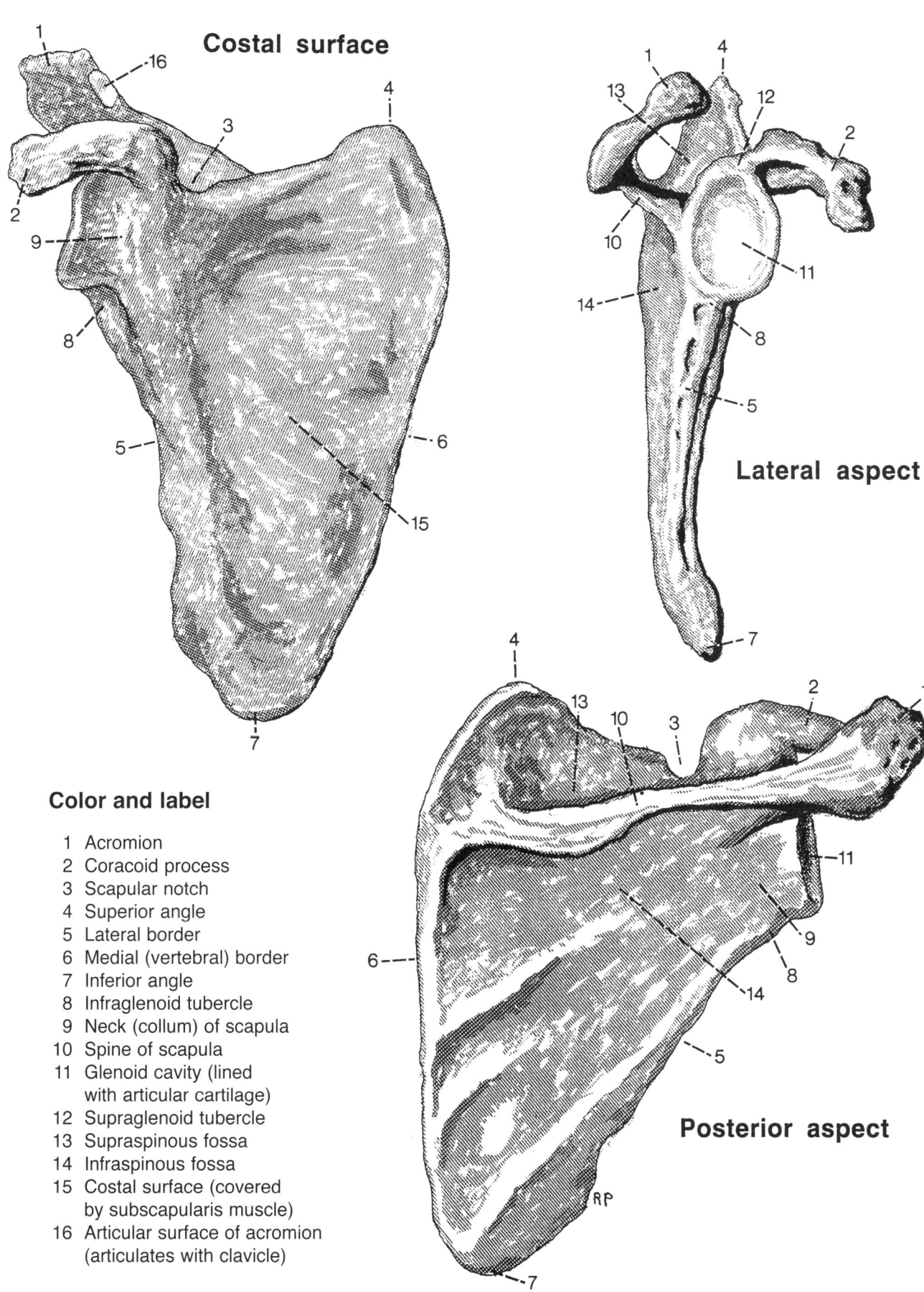

Color and label

1. Acromion
2. Coracoid process
3. Scapular notch
4. Superior angle
5. Lateral border
6. Medial (vertebral) border
7. Inferior angle
8. Infraglenoid tubercle
9. Neck (collum) of scapula
10. Spine of scapula
11. Glenoid cavity (lined with articular cartilage)
12. Supraglenoid tubercle
13. Supraspinous fossa
14. Infraspinous fossa
15. Costal surface (covered by subscapularis muscle)
16. Articular surface of acromion (articulates with clavicle)

Coracoid process and acromion (etymological cartoon)

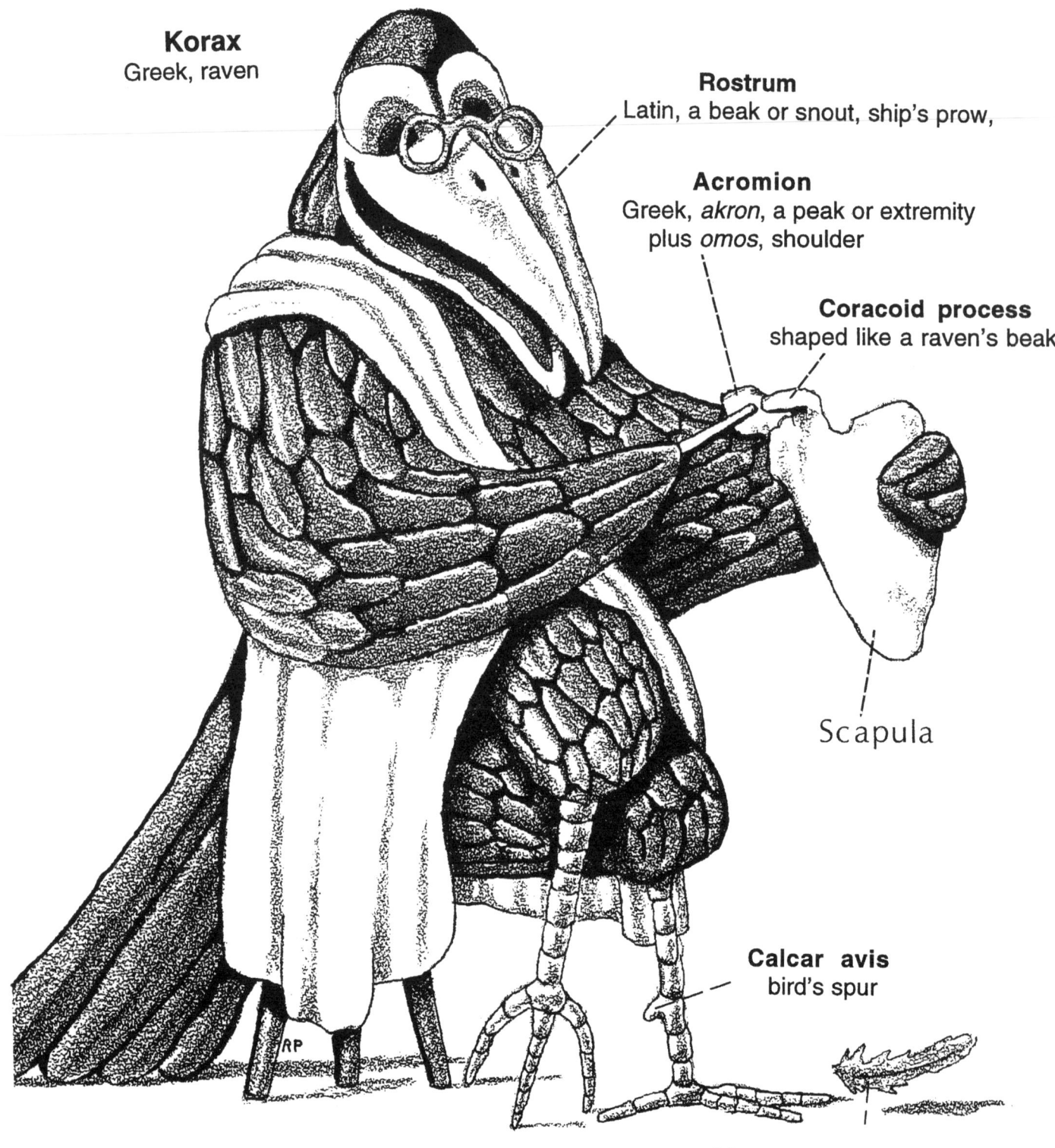

Korax
Greek, raven

Rostrum
Latin, a beak or snout, ship's prow,

Acromion
Greek, *akron*, a peak or extremity plus *omos*, shoulder

Coracoid process
shaped like a raven's beak

Scapula

Calcar avis
bird's spur

Pinna or penna
Latin, a feather, hence, our word *pen*

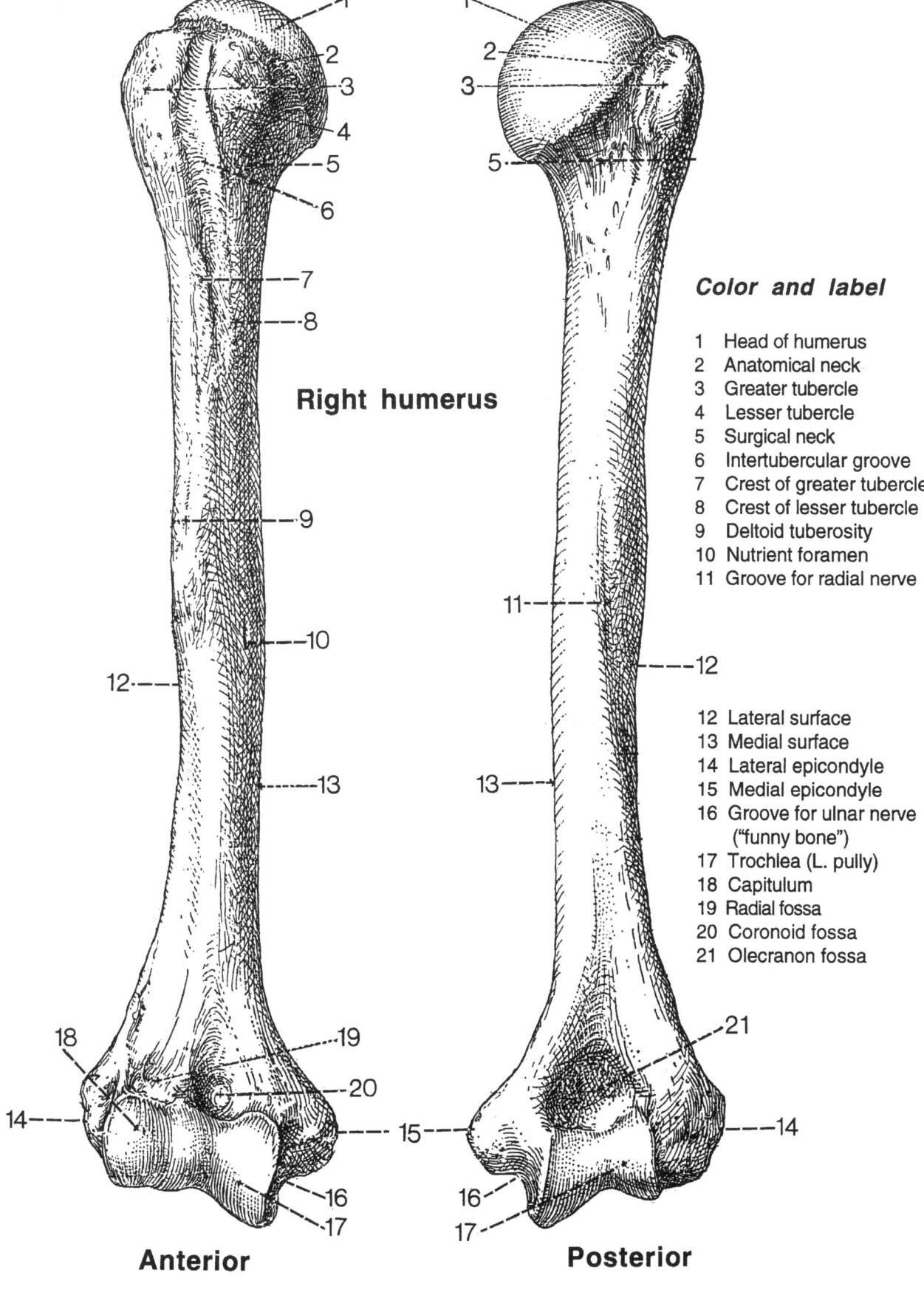

5 The radius and ulna

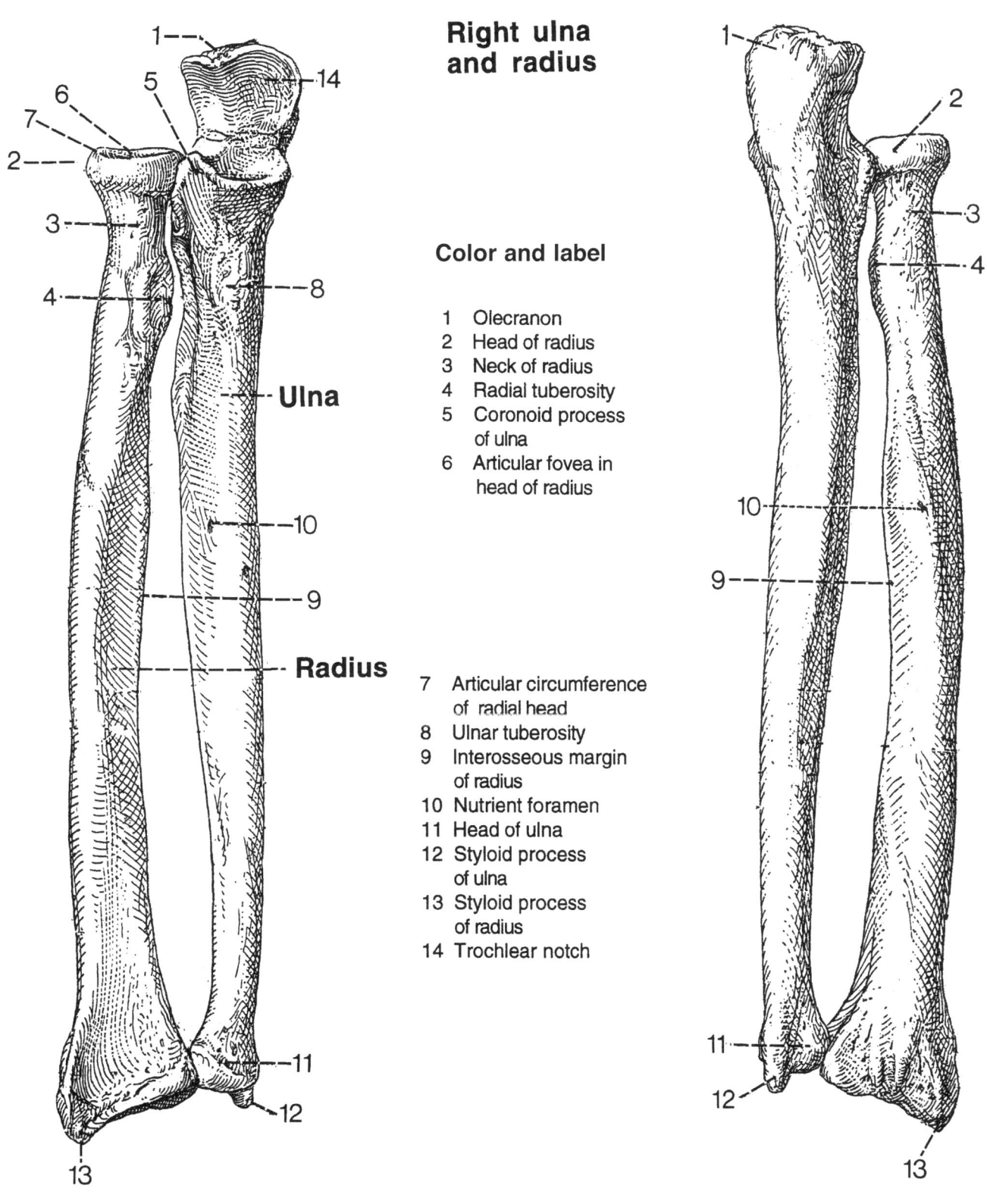

Right ulna and radius

Color and label

1. Olecranon
2. Head of radius
3. Neck of radius
4. Radial tuberosity
5. Coronoid process of ulna
6. Articular fovea in head of radius
7. Articular circumference of radial head
8. Ulnar tuberosity
9. Interosseous margin of radius
10. Nutrient foramen
11. Head of ulna
12. Styloid process of ulna
13. Styloid process of radius
14. Trochlear notch

Eycleshymer and Jones

6 Bones of the hand (manus)
Palmar aspect, right hand

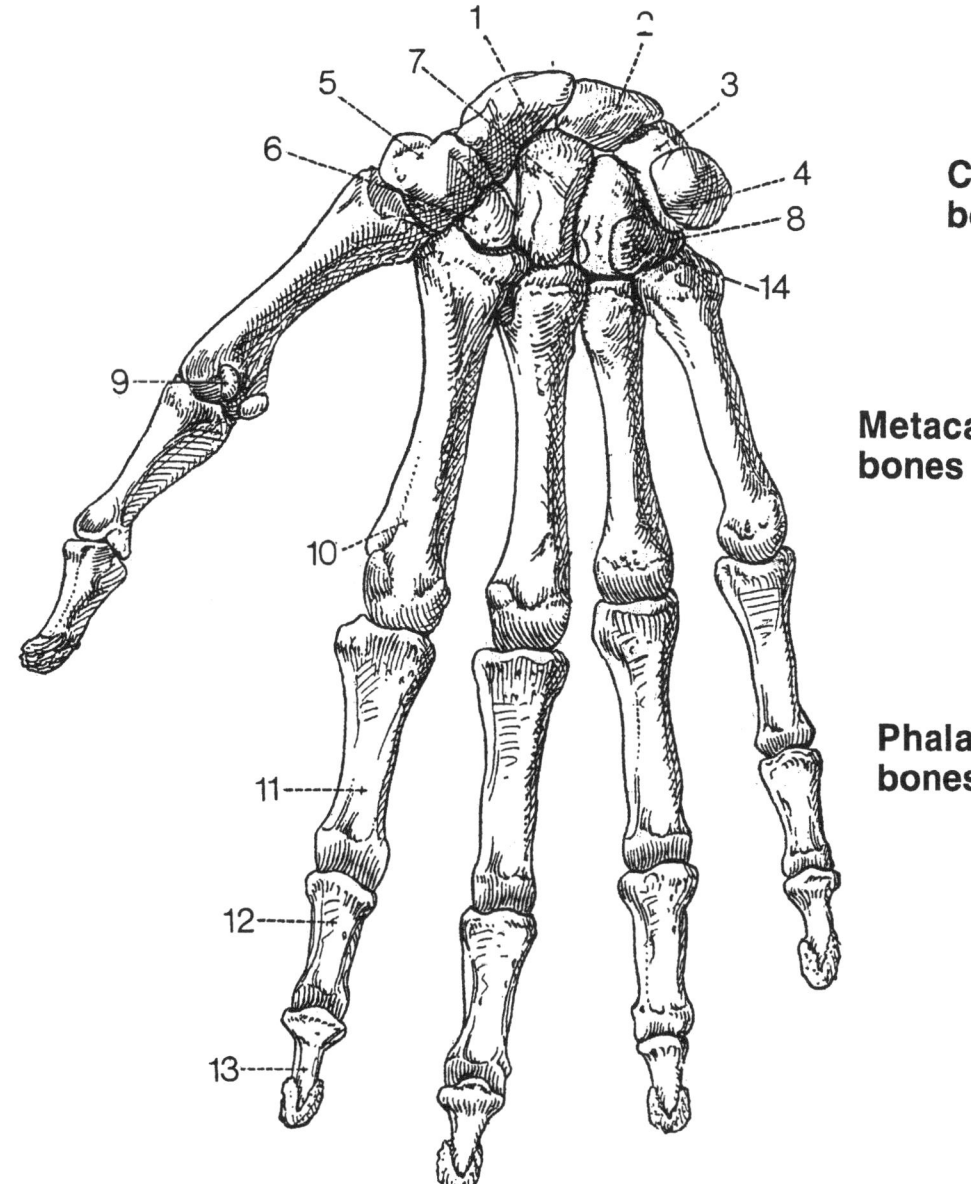

Carpal bones (8)
bones of the wrist

Metacarpal bones (5)
bones of the palm

Phalanges (14)
bones of the fingers

Eycleshymer and Jones

Color and label

1. Scaphoid (Gr. scapha, a hollowed-out small light boat)
2. Lunate (L. luna, the moon, moon-shaped)
3. Triquetral (three-sided)
4. Pisiform (L. pisum, a pea)
5. Trapezium (Gr. trapeza, a table)
6. Trapezoid (table-shaped)
7. Capitate (L. caput, head-shaped)
8. Hamate (hooked)
9. Sesamoid bones (resembling a sesame seed)
10. Second metacarpal bone
11. Proximal phalanx (second digit)
12. Middle phalanx
13. Distal phalanx
14. Hamulus of hamate (L. little hook)

7 Bones of the hand (manus)
Dorsal aspect, right hand

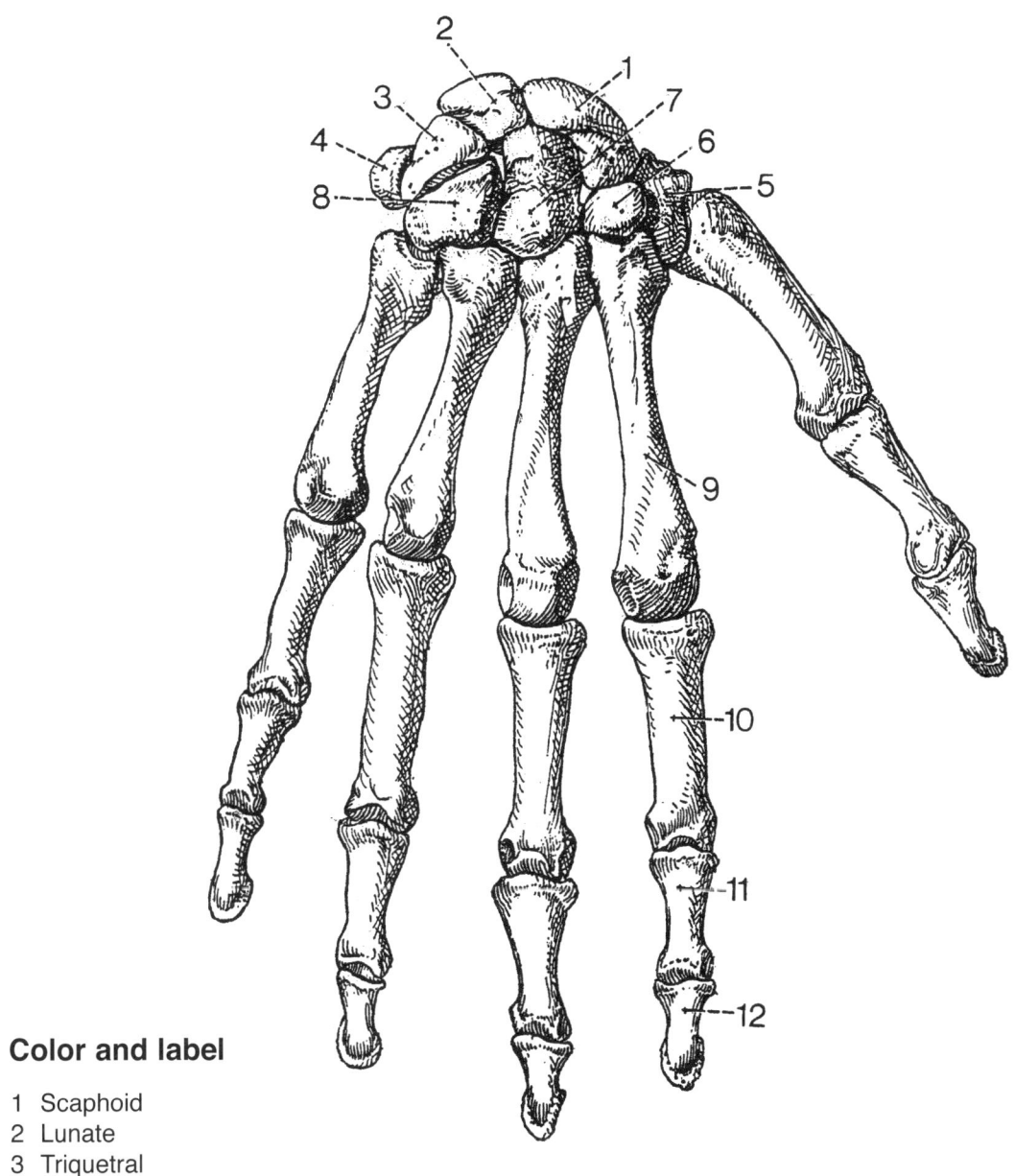

Color and label

1. Scaphoid
2. Lunate
3. Triquetral
4. Pisiform
5. Trapezium
6. Trapezoid
7. Capitate
8. Hamate
9. Second metacarpal
10. Proximal phalanx of index finger
11. Middle phalanx
12. Distal phalanx

Eycleshymer and Jones

Note that the thumb (L. pollex; combining form, pollicis), the most movable of the fingers, has only two phalanges, whereas the other four digits each have three phalanges.

8 Muscles of upper extremity I

Superficial muscles of right arm
Anterior view

Color and label

1. Clavicle
2. Trapezius (a small portion)
3. Pectoralis major
4. Coracobrachialis
5. Triceps brachii (long head)
6. Triceps brachii (medial head)
7. Brachialis
8. Pronator teres
9. Bicepital aponeurosis
10. Flexor carpi radialis
11. Palmaris longus
12. Flexor digitorum superficialis
13. Flexor carpi ulnaris
14. Pisiform bone
15. Flexor retinaculum
16. Palmaris brevis
17. Flexor pollicis brevis
18. Abductor pollicis brevis
19. Flexor pollicis longus
20. Flexor digitorum superficialis
21. Extensor carpi radialis longus
22. Extensor carpi radialis brevis
23. Brachioradialis
24. Biceps brachii tendon
25. Brachialis
26. Biceps brachii
27. Triceps brachii (lateral head)
28. Deltoid

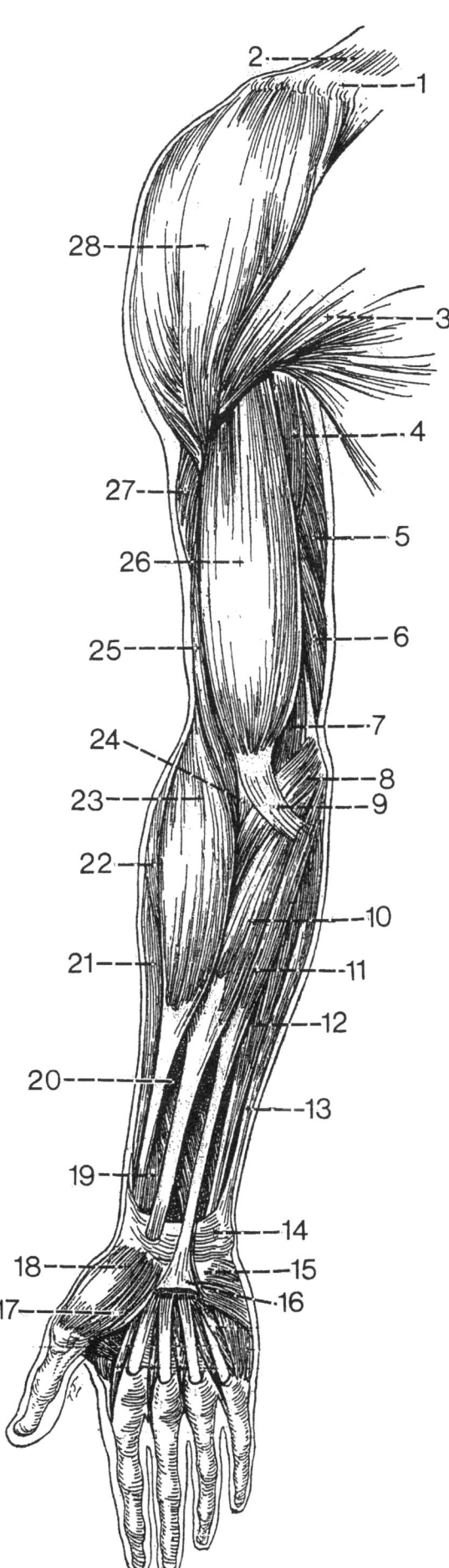

Eycleshymer and Jones

9 Muscles of upper extremity II

**Superficial muscles of right arm
Posterior view**

Color and label

1. Clavicle
2. Deltoid
3. Triceps brachii (lateral head)
4. Brachialis
5. Tendon of triceps brachii
6. Brachioradialis
7. Lateral epicondyle of humerus
8. Extensor carpi radialis longus
9. Extensor carpi radialis brevis
10. Abductor pollicis longus
11. Extensor pollicis brevis
12. Extensor pollicis longus
13. Tendon of extensor pollicis longus
14. Tendon of extensor pollicis brevis
15. Tendons of extensor digitorum
16. Extensor retinaculum
17. Extensor digiti minimi
18. Extensor digitorum
19. Extensor carpi ulnaris
20. Flexor carpi ulnaris
21. Anconeus
22. Olecranon
23. Medial epicondyle of humerus
24. Triceps brachii (medial head)
25. Triceps brachii (long head)

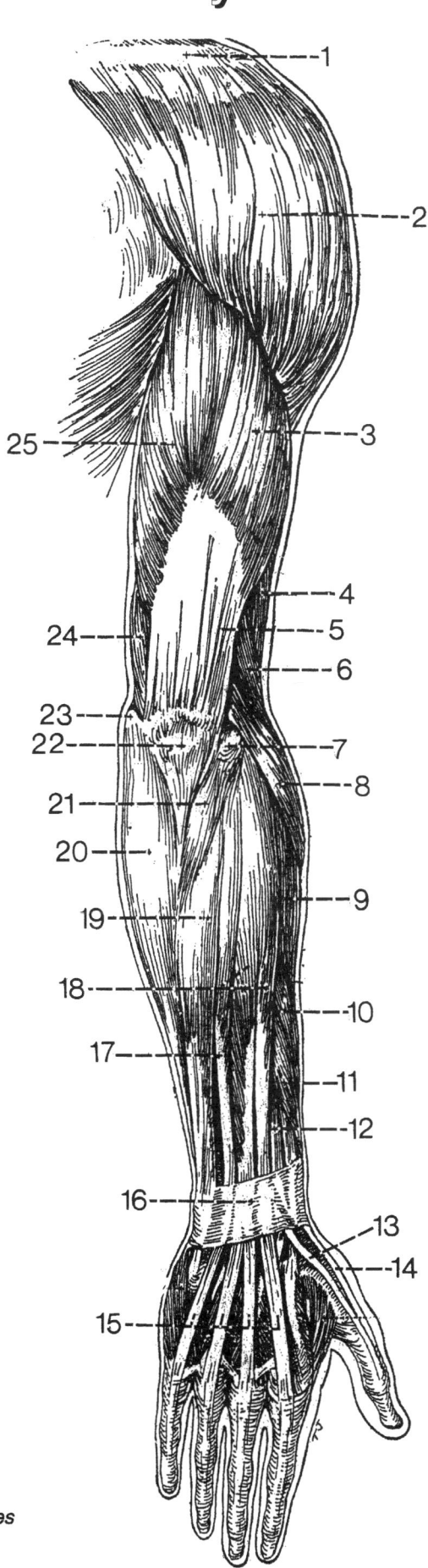

Eycleshymer and Jones

10 Muscles of upper extremity III

**Superficial muscles of right arm
Lateral view**

Color and label

1. Deltoid
2. Biceps brachii
3. Brachialis
4. Lateral intermuscular septum
5. Brachioradialis
6. Extensor carpi radialis longus
7. Extensor carpi radialis brevis
8. Abductor pollicis longus
9. Extensor pollicis brevis
10. Extensor retinaculum
11. "Snuff box"
12. Tendon of extensor pollicis longus
13. Tendon of extensor pollicis brevis
14. First dorsal interosseous
15. Tendons of extensor digitorum
16. Extensor digitorum
17. Extensor carpi ulnaris
18. Anconeus
19. Triceps brachii (lateral head)
20. Triceps brachii (long head)

Eycleshymer and Jones

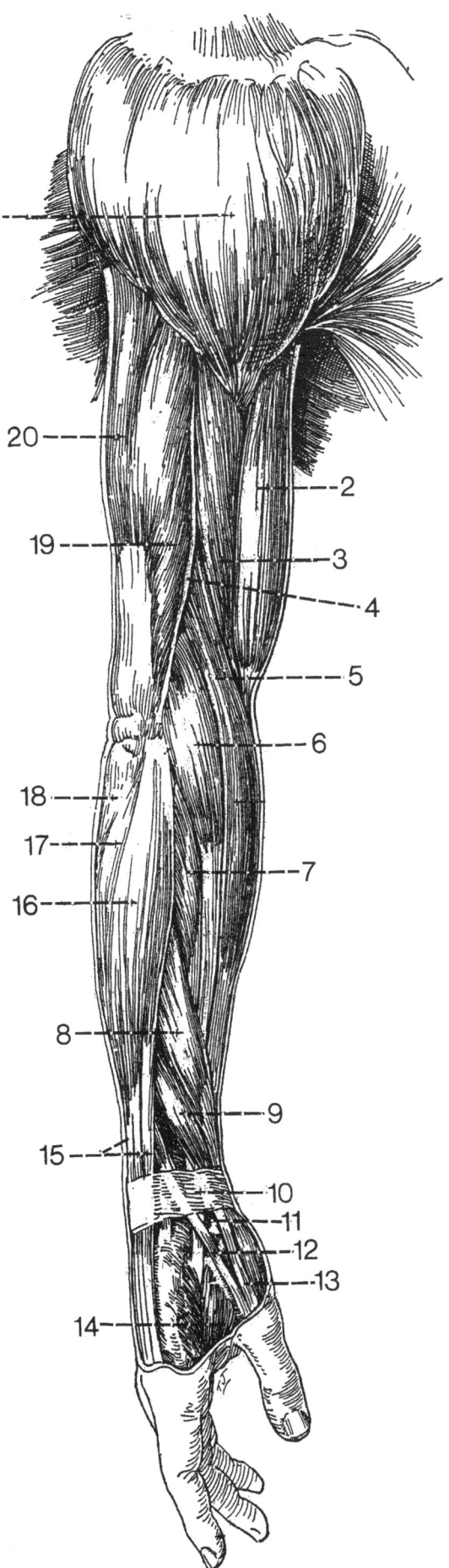

11 Dissection of posterior shoulder and arm

(opposite page)

Color and label

1 Accessory nerve; cranial nerve XI (old name, spinal accessory nerve). This nerve supplies two muscles, the trapezius and the sternocleidomastoid.
2 Trapezius muscle (upper fibers; cut)
3 Trapezius muscle - note its fibers insert on both the clavicle (26) and the spine of the scapula (10)
4 Trapezius (lower fibers); both sides of the trapezius together form a four-sided kite-shaped muscle.
5 Suprascapular nerve passing **through** the suprascapular foramen (notch) and **under** the transverse scapular ligament that bridges the suprascapular notch. The accompanying suprascapular artery and vein (not shown) pass **over** the transverse scapular ligament and **not through** the suprascapular foramen. The suprascapular nerve innervates the supraspinatus and infraspinatus muscles.
6 Axillary nerve passing backwards through the quadrangular space. It supplies the deltoid muscle and the teres minor muscle. Its branches form the upper lateral cutaneous nerve of the arm. It is accompanied by the posterior circumflex humeral artery and vein (not shown). The axillary nerve is one of the five major terminal branches of the brachial plexus.
7 Radial nerve. This nerve is the largest of the five terminal branches of the brachial plexus. It supplies all the extensor muscles in the upper limb including the three heads of the triceps, the brachioradialis, and the extensor digitorum. Here it winds posteriorly around the humerus in the radial groove accompanied by the profunda brachii artery (deep brachial artery) and vein (not shown). Its sensory fibers supply sensibility to most of the posterior surface of the upper limb.
8 Profunda brachii artery
9 Acromion process of scapula
10 Spine of scapula
11 Deltoid muscle (origin cut; arising on spine of scapula and acromion). It also arises from the lateral clavicle.
12 Deltoid muscle insertion on deltoid tuberosity of humerus
13 Deltoid muscle (cut in a coronal plane)
14 Supraspinatus muscle (cut)
15 Supraspinatus muscle (insertion on the superior facet of the greater tubercle of the humerus)
16 Infraspinatus muscle (cut)
17 Infraspinatus muscle (insertion on the middle facet of the greater tubercle of the humerus)
18 Teres minor muscle. The **rotator cuff** is formed by the subscapularis muscle anteriorly, the supraspinatus superiorly, and the infraspinatus and teres minor posteriorly.
19 Teres major muscle
20 Levator scapuli muscle
21 Rhomboid minor muscle
22 Rhomboid major muscle
23 Superficial branch of transverse cervical artery
24 Descending branch of superficial branch of transverse cervical artery
25 Deep branch of transverse cervical artery
26 Clavicle
27 Long head of triceps brachii
28 Lateral head of triceps brachii
29 Ascending branch of superficial branch of transverse cervical artery

11 Dissection of posterior shoulder and arm

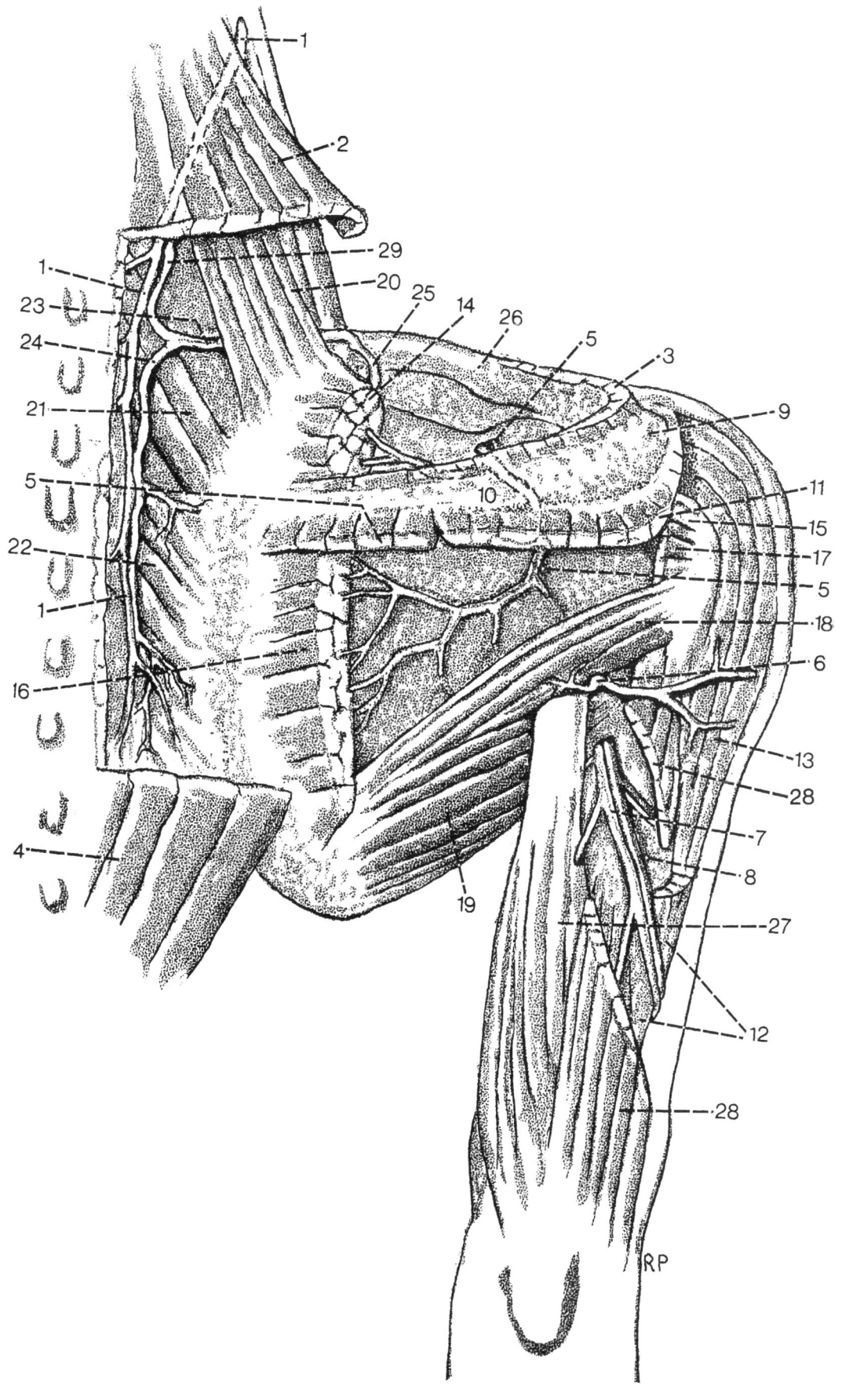

12 Nerves and arteries of the posterior shoulder

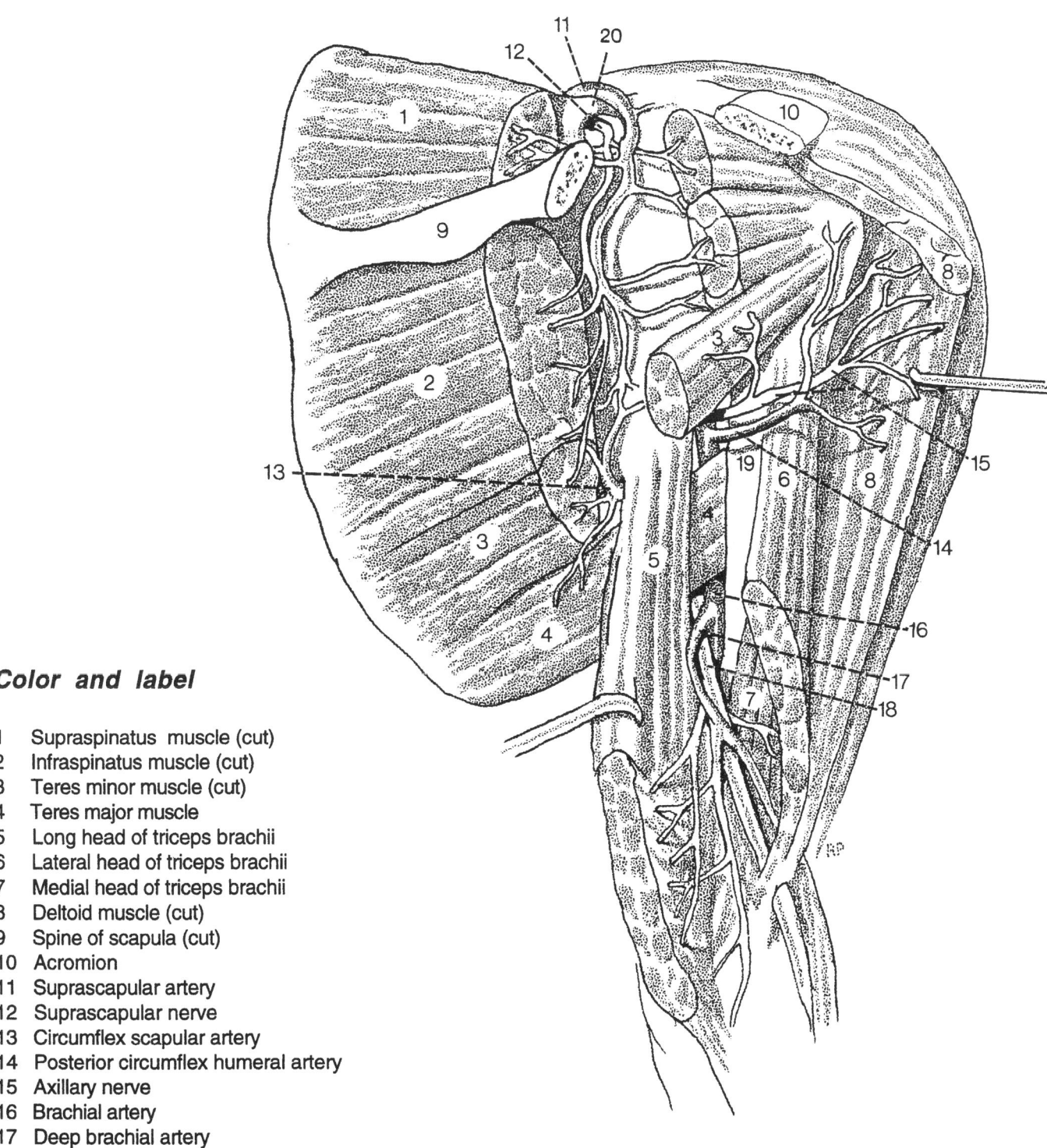

Color and label

1. Supraspinatus muscle (cut)
2. Infraspinatus muscle (cut)
3. Teres minor muscle (cut)
4. Teres major muscle
5. Long head of triceps brachii
6. Lateral head of triceps brachii
7. Medial head of triceps brachii
8. Deltoid muscle (cut)
9. Spine of scapula (cut)
10. Acromion
11. Suprascapular artery
12. Suprascapular nerve
13. Circumflex scapular artery
14. Posterior circumflex humeral artery
15. Axillary nerve
16. Brachial artery
17. Deep brachial artery
18. Radial nerve
19. Humerus
20. Transverse scapular ligament

After Wolf-Heidegger

13 Quadrangular space

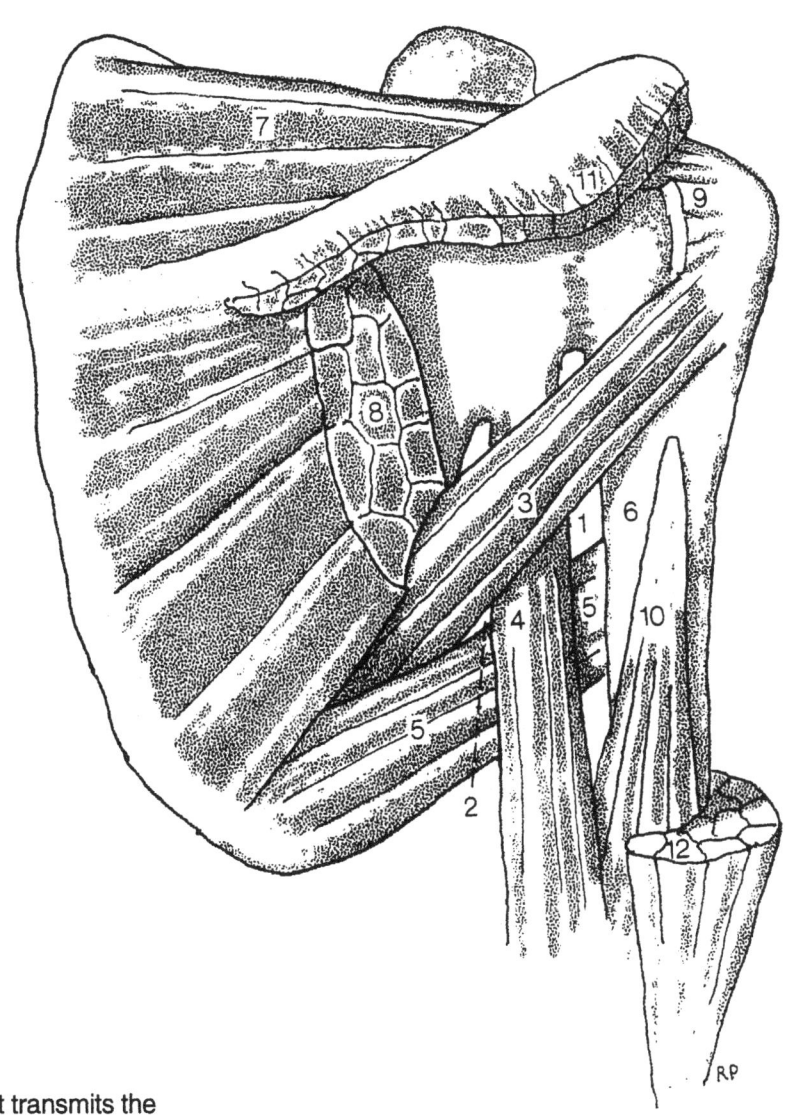

Color and label

1. Quadrangular space; it transmits the axillary nerve and the posterior circumflex humeral artery and vein
2. Triangular space
3. Teres minor (superior border of quadrangular space)
4. Long head of triceps brachii (medial border of space)
5. Teres major (inferior border of space)
6. Surgical neck of humerus (lateral border of space)
7. Supraspinatus muscle
8. Infraspinatus muscle
9. Insertion of infraspinatus muscle
10. Lateral head of triceps brachii
11. Origin of deltoid on spine and acromion of scapula
12. Deltoid muscle

14 The brachial plexus I
general plan

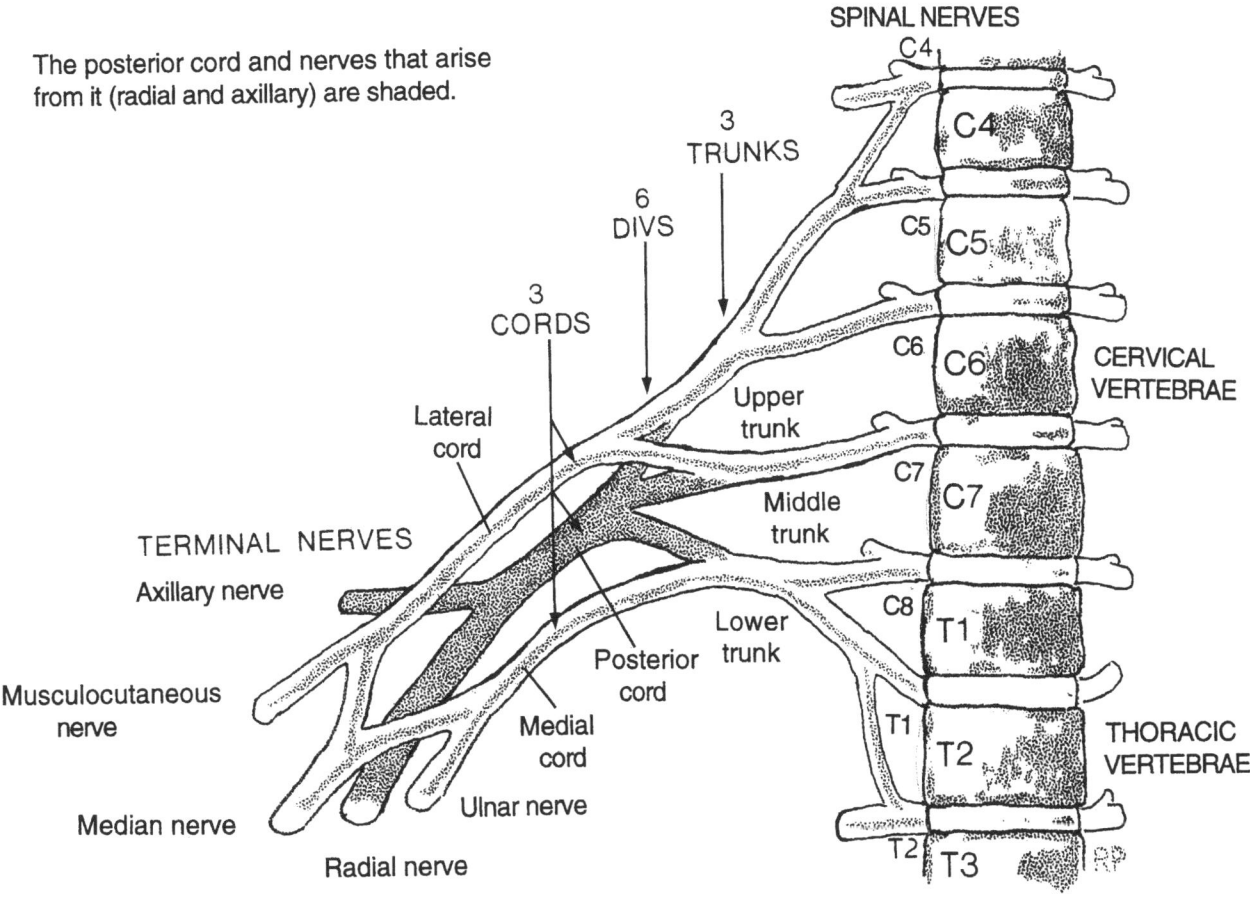

The **brachial plexus** supplies movement and sensation to the arm or upper extremity. It arises from spinal nerves in the neck. These nerves exchange nerve fibers (axons) by dividing and coalescing through five successive stages: nerves, trunks, divisions, cords, and terminal nerves. Beginning with cervical nerve C5 (with a contribution from cervical nerve C4) down to thoracic nerve T1 (with a contribution from T2) they fuse into three trunks (an upper, middle, and lower trunk); each trunk then divides into an anterior and a posterior division resulting in six divisions; the six divisions coalesce into three cords which then give off five large terminal nerves, the radial nerve, the axillary nerve, the median nerve, the musculocutaneous nerve, and the ulnar nerve. (See following figure for additional nerves that are given off by the brachial plexus.)

Note that there are 8 cervical nerves but only 7 cervical vertebrae. Cervical nerves 1-7 exit the vertebral column **above** the corresponding vertebra (cervical nerve C7 exits **above** cervical vertebra C7), whereas cervical nerve C8 exits **below** vertebra C7. All susequent (lower) spinal nerves (thoracic and lumbar) exit below their corresponding vertebrae.

15 Brachial plexus and its nerves II
(opposite page)

Color and label

1   Phrenic nerve. The motor nerve to the diaphragm. It arises from branches of cervical nerves C3, C4, and C5. It passes inferiorly in front of the root of the lung, pierces the diaphragm and innervates it on its inferior surface.
2   Dorsal scapular nerve. A branch of the fifth cervical nerve. It pierces the scalenus medius muscle and reaches the deep surface of the rhomboids which it supplies and sometimes the levator scapulae.
3   Suprascapular nerve. A branch (with fibers from C5 and C6) of the superior trunk. It supplies the supraspinatus and infraspinatus muscles after passing backwards under the ligament that bridges the suprascapular notch.
4   Nerve to the subclavius muscle. A branch (C5,C6) of the superior trunk.
5   Upper trunk of brachial plexus
6   Lateral pectoral nerve. A branch (C5-C7) of the lateral cord supplying the clavicular and upper sternal portion of the pectoralis major muscle. Some of its fibers reach the pectoralis minor muscle through a communicating link (7) with the medial pectoral nerve.
7   Communicating link between the lateral and medial pectoral nerves
8   Lateral cord of brachial plexus
9   Musculocutaneous nerve. A major terminal branch (C5-C7) of the brachial plexus that innervates the flexor muscles of the upper arm, coracobrachialis (which it penetrates), the biceps brachii, and the brachialis. It emerges in the forearm as the lateral cutaneous nerve which supplies the skin of the lateral (radial) forearm as far as the thenar eminence. Hence its name, the "muscle-skin" nerve.
10 Lateral root of median nerve
11 Median nerve. A major nerve (C5-T1) to the flexor muscles of the forearm and hand. It supplies sensation to the radial 3 1/2 digits (including the thumb) plus motor fibers to the critically important thumb muscles, the abductor pollicis brevis, the flexor pollicis brevis, and the opponens pollicis. In the forearm it gives rise to the anterior interosseous nerve.
12 Medial root of the median nerve
13 Ulnar nerve. A major terminal nerve arising from the medial cord of the brachial plexus. As it passes superficially over the medial epicondyle of the humerus it is vulnerable to an external tap which is usually felt as the instantaneous painful " funny bone" sensation. It suppies the skin of the front and back of the medial hand, most of the small muscles in the hand, plus some flexor muscles in the forearm.
14 Radial nerve. The largest terminal nerve (C5-C8) of the brachial plexus. It supplies all the extensor muscles of the upper limb. Its cutaneous branches supply sensibility to the dorsal surface of the upper limb from the insertion of the deltoid to the dorsum of the wrist. It supplies the long forearm extensor and abductor muscles to the digits, but it supplies no intrinsic hand muscles.
15 Axillary nerve. A major terminal branch of the brachial plexus. It carries axons from cervicle nerves C5 and C6. It leaves the posterior cord and passes backwards through the quadrangular space to innervate the deltoid and teres minor muscles.
16 Medial cord of brachial plexus
17 Medial antebrachial cutaneous nerve (C8,T1). Supplies sensibility to the skin of the medial forearm.
18 Medial brachial cutaneous nerve (C8,T1). Supplies the skin of the medial (upper) arm.
19 Medial pectoral nerve. Innervates the pectoralis major and minor muscles.
20 Posterior cord of brachial plexus
21 Inferior subscapular nerve. Innervates caudal portion of subscapularis muscle and teres major muscle.
22 Thoracodorsal nerve (also middle subscapular nerve). Arises from the posterior cord. It suppies the latissimus dorsi muscle.
23 Superior subscapular nerve. Innervates cranial portion of subscapularis muscle
24 Anterior and posterior divisions of the 3 trunks of the brachial plexus (6 in all)
25 Middle trunk of the brachial plexus
26 Lower trunk of the brachial plexus
27 Long thoracic nerve to the serratus anterior muscle
28 Nerves to prevertebral muscles and scalene muscles

15 Brachial plexus and its nerves II

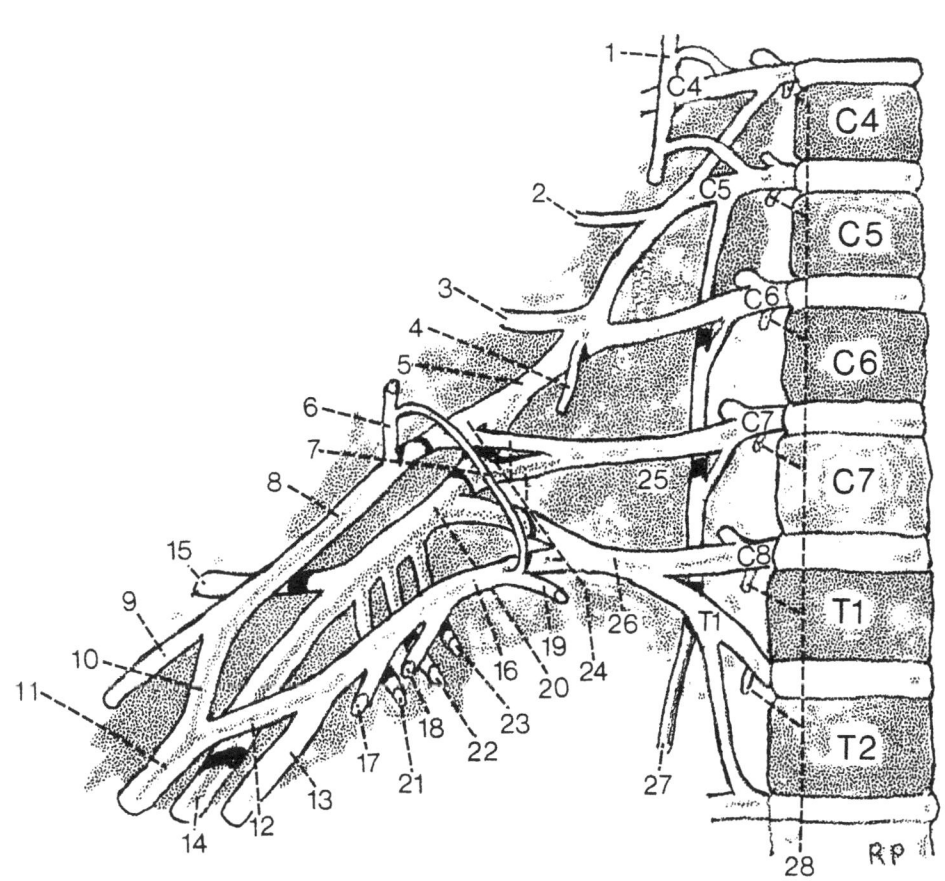

16 Arteries of the posterior shoulder and arm
(opposite page)

Color and label

SC-1 First part of subclavian artery; the major artery to the upper extremity; the right subclavian artery begins at the bifurcation of the brachiocephalic trunk into the right subclavian and right common carotid arteries. The left subclavian and common carotid arteries originate from the convexity of the aortic arch.
SC-2 Second part of subclavian artery (behind anterior scalene muscle)
SC-3 Third part of subclavian artery (continues as the axillary in the shoulder)

1 Brachiocephalic trunk (old name, innominate artery)
2 Common carotid artery (the left common carotid arises from the convexity of the aortic arch)
3 Right vagus nerve
4 Recurrent laryngeal nerve (branch of the vagus nerve)
5 Vertebral artery
6 Thyrocervical trunk (origin on ventral side of subclavian artery) (see insert on upper right)
7 Inferior thyroid artery
8 Ascending cervical artery
9 Transverse cervical artery
10 Superficial branch of transverse cervical artery (supplies trapezius)
11 Ascending branch of (10)
12 Descending branch of (10); It lies deep to trapezius but superficial to rhomboids.
13 Deep branch of transverse cervical artery (it accompanies dorsal scapular nerve)
14 Dorsal scapular nerve (a small section)
15 Suprascapular artery (passes over the transverse scapular ligament)
16 Suprascapular nerve (passes under transverse scapular ligament)
17 Arterial plexus within supraspinatus muscle (not shown)
18 Arterial plexus within infraspinatus muscle (not shown)
19 Axillary artery (continuation of subclavian artery)
20 Internal thoracic artery (old name, internal mammary artery)
21 Costocervical trunk
22 Supreme (or highest) intercostal artery
23 Deep cervical artery
24 Subscapular artery
25 Circumflex scapular artery
26 Thoracodorsal artery
27 Posterior circumflex humeral artery (passes through quadrangular space)
28 Anterior circumflex humeral artery
29 Brachial artery (continuation of axillary artery)
30 Deep brachial artery (profunda brachii artery)
31 Deltoid artery (ascending branch)
32 Superior ulnar collateral artery
33 Inferior ulnar collateral artery
34 Posterior ulnar recurrent artery
35 Radial collateral branch of deep brachial artery
36 Middle collateral branch of deep brachial artery
37 Ulnar artery
38 Radial artery
39 Common interosseous artery (a short thick branch of ulnar artery; divides into anterior and posterior interosseous arteries)
40 Posterior interosseous artery
41 Anterior interosseous artery
42 Recurrent interosseous artery (it may arise from the common interosseous artery)
43 Axillary nerve (cut)
44 Radial nerve (cut)
45 Ulnar nerve (a small section)

16 Arteries of the posterior shoulder and arm

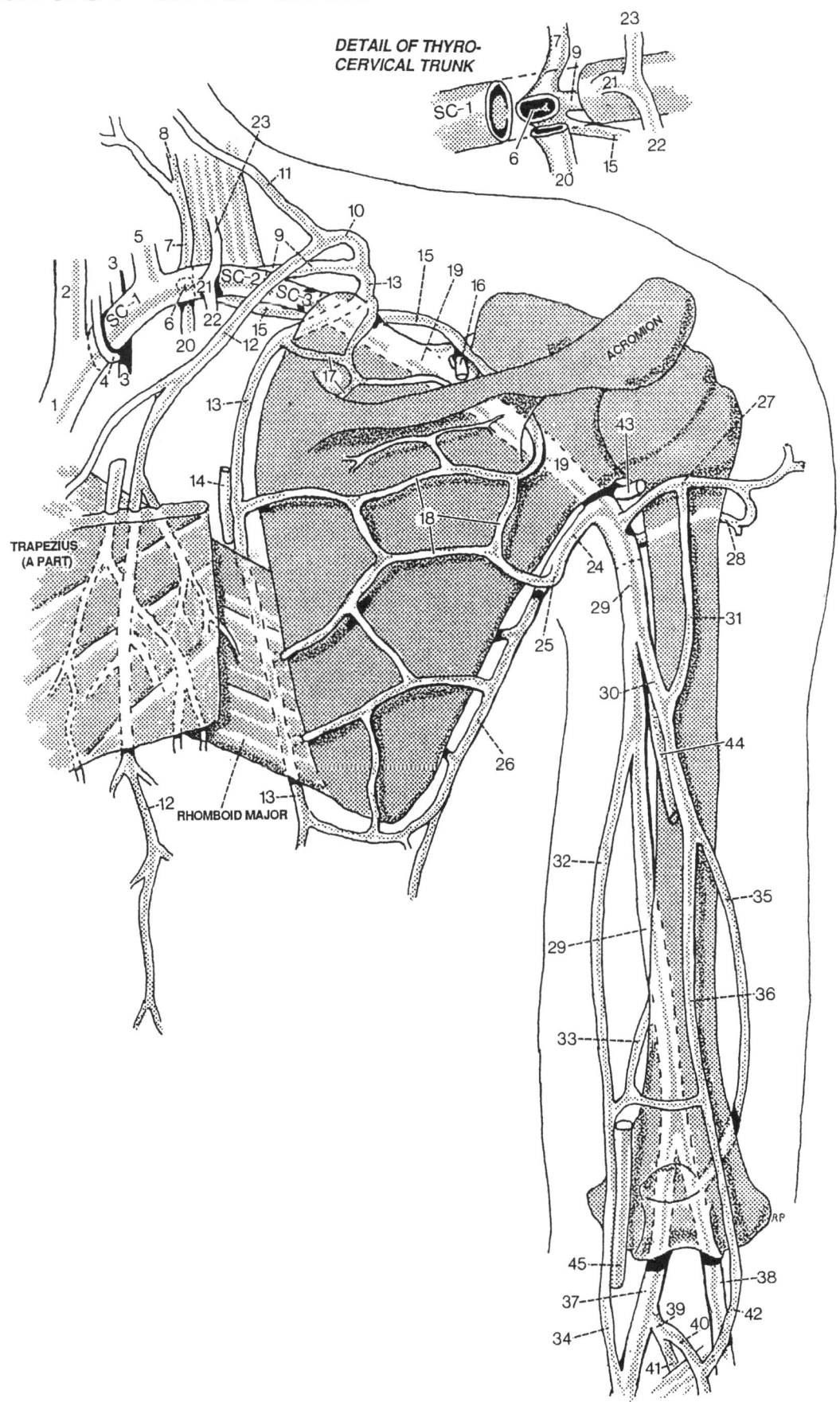

17 Subclavian artery, axillary artery, and brachial artery (opposite page)

Viewed from the front (anterior aspect)

Color and label

1 Ascending aorta (behind sternum and manubrium)
2 Brachiocephalic trunk
3 Left common carotid artery
4 Right common carotid artery
5 Subclavian artery
6 Vertebral artery
7 Thyrocervical trunk
8 Inferior thyroid artery
9 Ascending cervical artery
10 Inferior layngeal artery
11 Transverse cervical artery
12 Superficial branch of transverse cervical artery
13 Deep branch of transverse cervical artery
14 Ascending branch of superficial branch of transverse cervical artery
15 Descending branch of superficial branch of transverse cervical artery
16 Suprascapular artery
17 Internal thoracic (mammary) artery
18 Anterior intercostal arteries (the intercostal arteries are accompanied by intercostal veins and intercostal nerves; not shown here)
19 Perforating branches
20 Musculophrenic artery (terminal branch of the internal thoracic artery)
21 Superior epigastric artery (terminal branch of the internal thoracic artery)
22 Deep cervical artery
23 Axillary artery
24 Supreme thoracic artery
25 Thoracoacromial trunk
26 Clavicular branch of (25)
27 Acromial branch of (25)
28 Deltoid branch of (25)
29 Pectoral branches of (25)
30 Lateral thoracic artery (may also arise from thoracoacromial trunk or from subscapular artery)
31 Subscapular artery
32 Circumflex scapular artery
33 Thoracodorsal artery
34 Anterior humeral circumflex artery
35 Posterior humeral circumflex artery
36 Brachial artery
37 Deep brachial artery
38 Radial collateral artery (of deep brachial artery)
39 Middle collateral artery (of deep brachial artery)
40 Superior ulnar collateral artery
41 Inferior ulnar collateral artery
42 Anterior ulnar recurrent artery
43 Posterior ulnar recurrent artery
44 Radial recurrent artery
45 Interosseous recurrent artery
46 Posterior interosseous artery
47 Anterior interosseous artery
48 Common interosseous artery

The dissector should understand that, with very few exceptions, veins (not shown here) accompany arteries. The veins may be single or double and tend to be more irregular in their pattern than arteries. One should expect to encounter variations in the pattern of both arteries and veins that differ from the figures depicted here.

17 Subclavian artery, axillary artery, and brachial artery

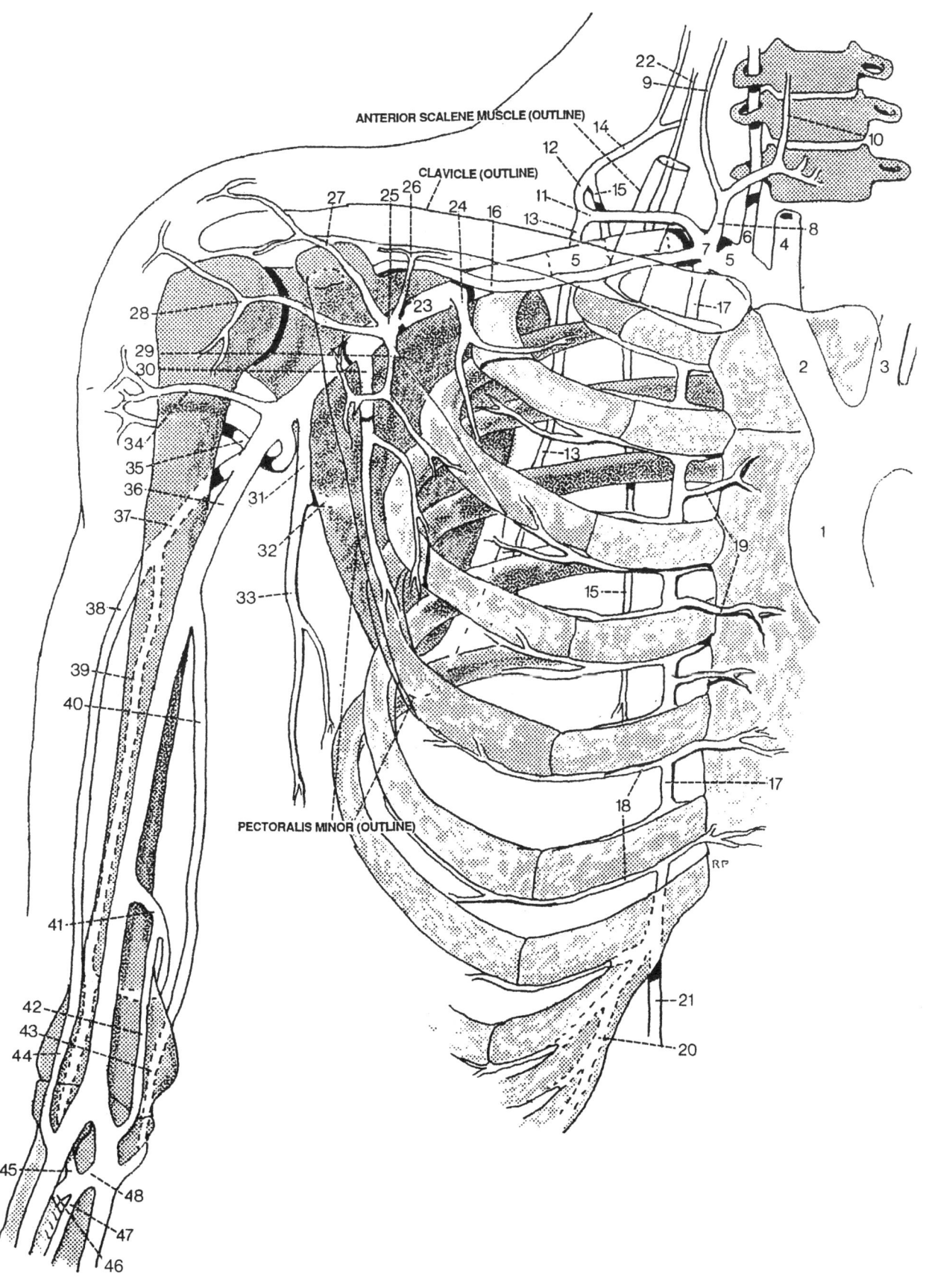

18 Superficial veins and nerves of the anterior arm

Right arm, anterior surface

Color and label

1. Palmar (volar) digital veins
2. Superficial palmar venous arch
3. Intermediate antebrachial vein
4. Basilic vein
5. Cephalic vein
6. Intermediate cubital vein (old name, median cubital)
7. Intermediate basilic vein
8. Accessory cephalic vein
9. Medial brachial cutaneous nerve (branches)
10. Medial antebrachial cutaneous nerve
11. Lateral antebrachial cutaneous nerve (musculocutaneous nerve)
12. Palmar branch of median nerve
13. Palmar branch of ulnar nerve
14. Posterior antebrachial cutaneous nerve (radial nerve)
15. Superficial branch of radial nerve

Eycleshymer and Jones

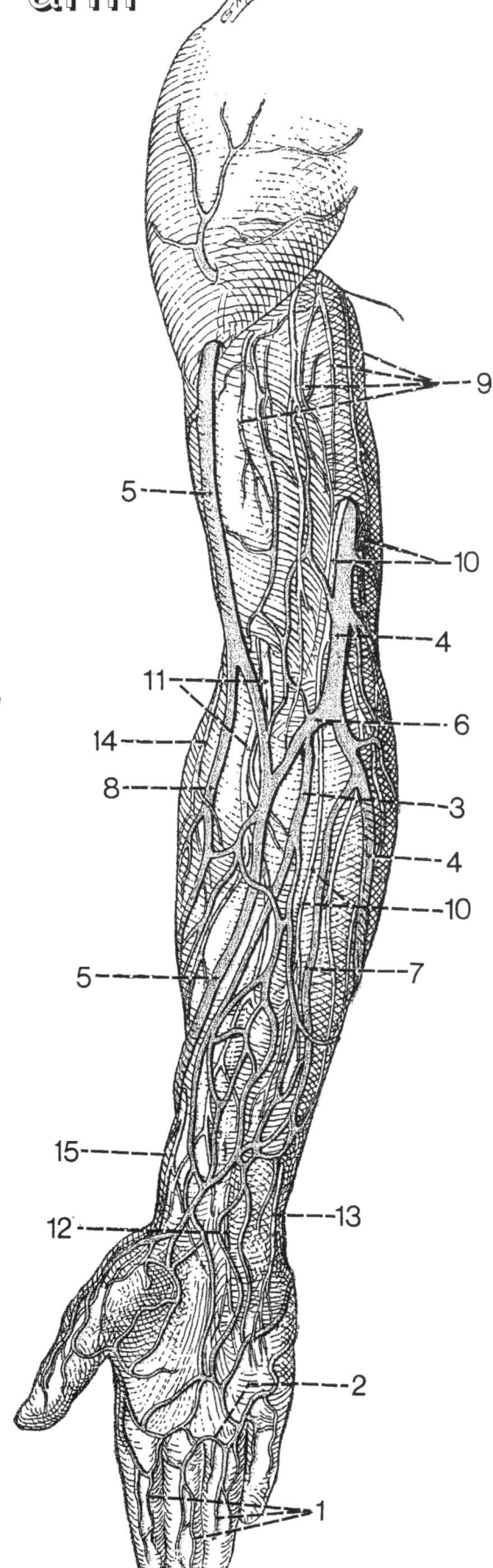

19 Superficial veins and nerves of the posterior arm

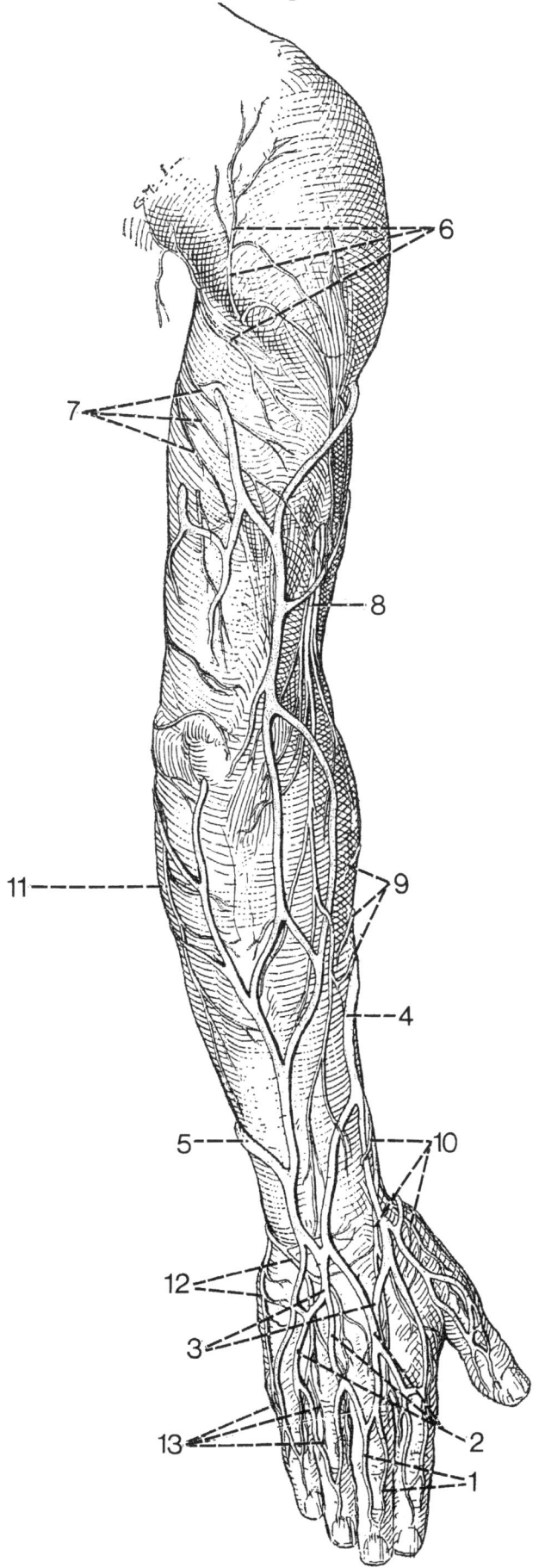

Right arm, posterior surface

Color and label

1. Dorsal digital veins
2. Dorsal metacarpal veins
3. Dorsal venous network of the hand
4. Cephalic vein
5. Basilic vein
6. Lateral superior brachial cutaneous nerve (of axillary nerve)
7. Posterior brachial cutaneous nerve (of radial nerve)
8. Posterior antebrachial cutaneous nerve (of radial nerve)
9. Lateral antebrachial cutaneous nerve (of musculocutaneous nerve)
10. Superficial branch of radial nerve
11. Medial antebrachial cutaneous nerve
12. Branch of ulnar nerve to dorsum of the hand
13. Dorsal digital nerves

Eycleshymer and Jones

20 Deep dissection of the posterior arm

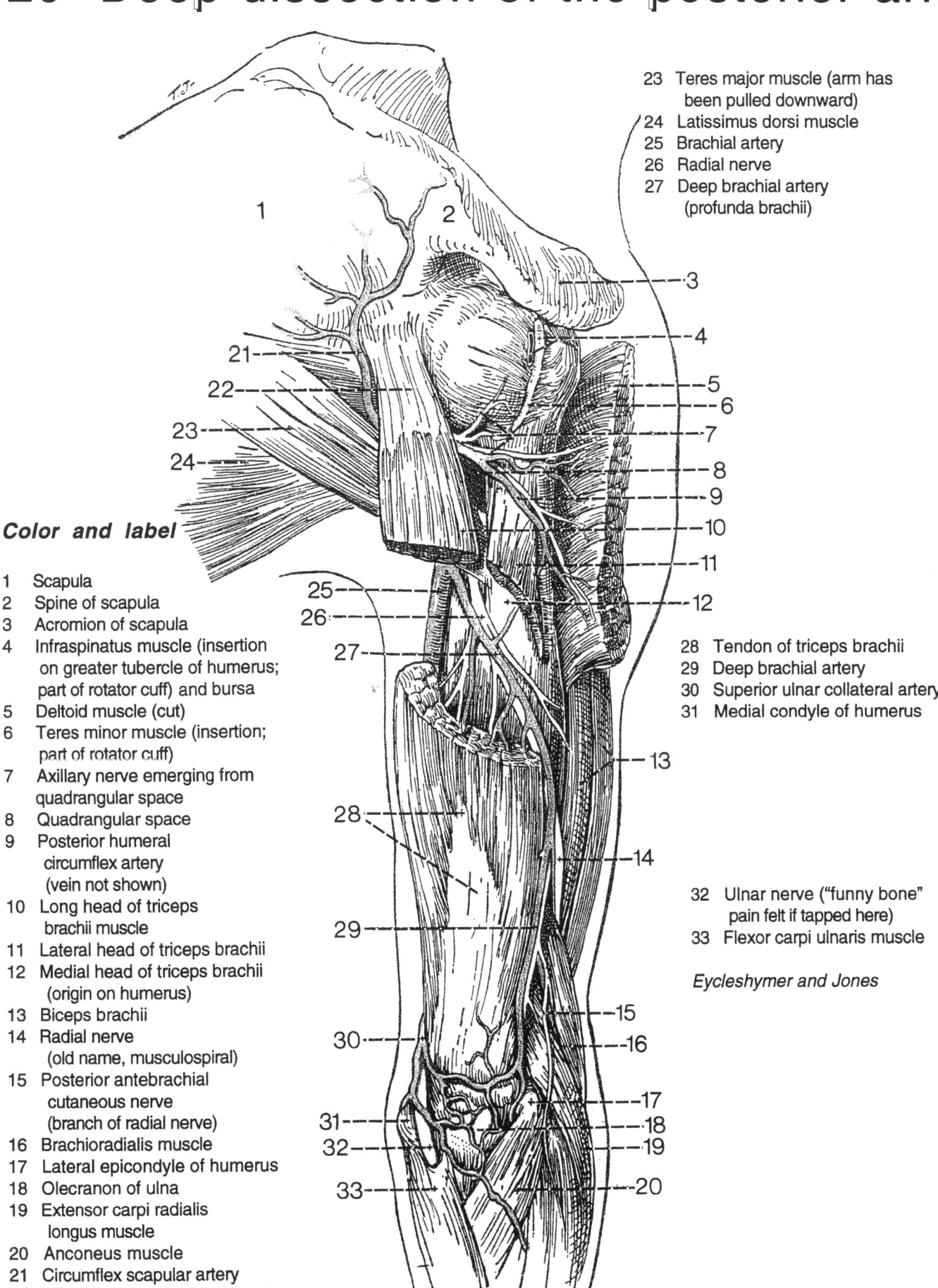

Color and label

1. Scapula
2. Spine of scapula
3. Acromion of scapula
4. Infraspinatus muscle (insertion on greater tubercle of humerus; part of rotator cuff) and bursa
5. Deltoid muscle (cut)
6. Teres minor muscle (insertion; part of rotator cuff)
7. Axillary nerve emerging from quadrangular space
8. Quadrangular space
9. Posterior humeral circumflex artery (vein not shown)
10. Long head of triceps brachii muscle
11. Lateral head of triceps brachii
12. Medial head of triceps brachii (origin on humerus)
13. Biceps brachii
14. Radial nerve (old name, musculospiral)
15. Posterior antebrachial cutaneous nerve (branch of radial nerve)
16. Brachioradialis muscle
17. Lateral epicondyle of humerus
18. Olecranon of ulna
19. Extensor carpi radialis longus muscle
20. Anconeus muscle
21. Circumflex scapular artery (branch of subscapular artery)
22. Long head of triceps brachii
23. Teres major muscle (arm has been pulled downward)
24. Latissimus dorsi muscle
25. Brachial artery
26. Radial nerve
27. Deep brachial artery (profunda brachii)
28. Tendon of triceps brachii
29. Deep brachial artery
30. Superior ulnar collateral artery
31. Medial condyle of humerus
32. Ulnar nerve ("funny bone" pain felt if tapped here)
33. Flexor carpi ulnaris muscle

Eycleshymer and Jones

21 Brachial plexus III (opposite page)

Color and label

1. Upper trunk
2. Middle trunk
3. Lower trunk
4. Lateral cord. It continues mainly as the musculocutaneous nerve. Carries fibers from spinal nerves C5, C6, C7.
5. Posterior cord; the posterior cord receives nerve fibers from spinal nerves C5-T1 by way of all 3 posterior divisions; two large nerves arise from the posterior cord, the radial nerve and the axillary nerve.
6. Medial cord; its nerve fibers continue mainly as the ulnar nerve. Carries fibers from C8 and T1. The 3 cords are named by their relation to the axillary artery, lateral, posterior, and medial.
7. Musculocutaneous nerve. It is the main continuation of the lateral cord with fibers from spinal nerves C5, C6, C7. It penetrates the coracobrachialis muscle which it supplies along with the biceps brachii and the brachialis.
8. Median nerve. Contains fibers from spinal nerves C5,C6,C7,C8, T1. It is formed by two roots, a lateral root from the lateral cord and a medial root from the medial cord. Note how these two roots plus the musculocutaneous nerve and the ulnar nerve form an "M". This "M" formation may occur further distally.
9. Ulnar nerve (C8,T1)
10. Radial nerve (C5,C6,C7,C8,T1)
11. Axillary nerve (C5,C6)
12. Brachial artery
13. Subclavian artery. This becomes the axillary artery at the lateral border of the first rib.
14. Dashed outline of the axillary artery (rendered transparent to show the posterior cord). Note that the posterior cord is directly posterior to the axillary artery. The axillary artery becomes the brachial artery at the lower border of the teres major.
15. Dashed outline of the brachial artery.
16. Dorsal scapular nerve to rhomboid major and minor
17. Nerve to subclavius
18. Long thoracic nerve to serratus anterior
19. Suprascapular nerve to supraspinatus and infraspinatus
20. Medial pectoral nerve
21. Lateral pectoral nerve
22. Subscapular nerve to subscapularis and teres major
23. Medial cutaneous nerve of forearm (medial antebrachial cutaneous nerve)
24. Medial cutaneous nerve of (upper) arm (medial brachial cutaneous nerve)
25. Humerus
26. Short head of biceps brachii
27. Coracobrachialis
28. Pectoralis minor (cut)
29. Clavicle (rendered partly transparent)
30. Latissimus dorsi
31. Right common carotid artery
32. Scalenus anterior. This muscle divides the subclavian artery into 3 parts: first part medial to the muscle; second part behind the muscle; third part lateral to the muscle.

21 Brachial plexus III

Redrawn from Gray's Anatomy, 38th British ed., P.L. Williams, editor, Edinburgh, Churchill Livingstone, 1995

22 Nerves of the upper right limb
(opposite page)
Anterior aspect

Color and label

1. Axillary artery
2. Lateral cord of brachial plexus
3. Medial cord of brachial plexus
4. Median nerve; note its formation by two roots, one from the lateral cord and one from the medial cord.
5. Ulnar nerve
6. Musculocutaneous nerve; after penetrating and supplying the coracobrachialis muscle, it continues on to innervate the biceps brachii and brachialis.
7. Radial nerve (superficial branch)
8. Lateral antebrachial cutaneous nerve (lateral cutaneous nerve of forearm)
9. Anterior interosseous nerve
10. Brachial artery; the axillary artery becomes the brachial artery at the inferior border of the teres major.
11. Ulnar artery
12. Radial artery
13. Median nerve entering palm after emerging from under the flexor retinaculum
14. Branch of median nerve to thenar (thumb) muscles
15. Lateral pectoral nerve; it innervates both the pectoralis major and pectoralis minor; note its connection to the medial pectoral nerve.
16. Medial pectoral nerve; after entering and innervating the pectoralis minor, it continues on to supply the costal and lower sternal portions of the pectoralis major.
17. Long thoracic nerve; it supplies the serratus anterior muscle.
18. Intercostobrachial nerve. This is the lateral cutaneous branch of the second thoracic nerve; note its joining the medial brachial cutaneous nerve (19) with which it supplies the skin of the medial (upper) arm.
19. Medial brachial cutaneous nerve
20. Medial antebrachial cutaneous nerve
21. Deltoid muscle
22. Tendon of pectoralis minor (cut)
23. Pectoralis major muscle
24. Pectoralis minor muscle
25. Short head of biceps brachii
26. Long head of biceps brachii
27. Tendon of pectoralis major muscle (cut)
28. Coracobrachialis muscle
29. Brachialis muscle
30. Biceps brachii muscle
31. Pronator teres (superficial head)(cut)
32. Pronator teres (deep head); note the median nerve passes between the two heads of the pronator teres.
33. Brachioradialis muscle
34. Flexor carpi ulnaris muscle
35. Flexor pollicis longus tendon
36. Tendon of palmaris longus (cut)
37. Flexor retinaculum
38. Serratus anterior muscle

22 Nerves of the upper right limb

Anterior aspect

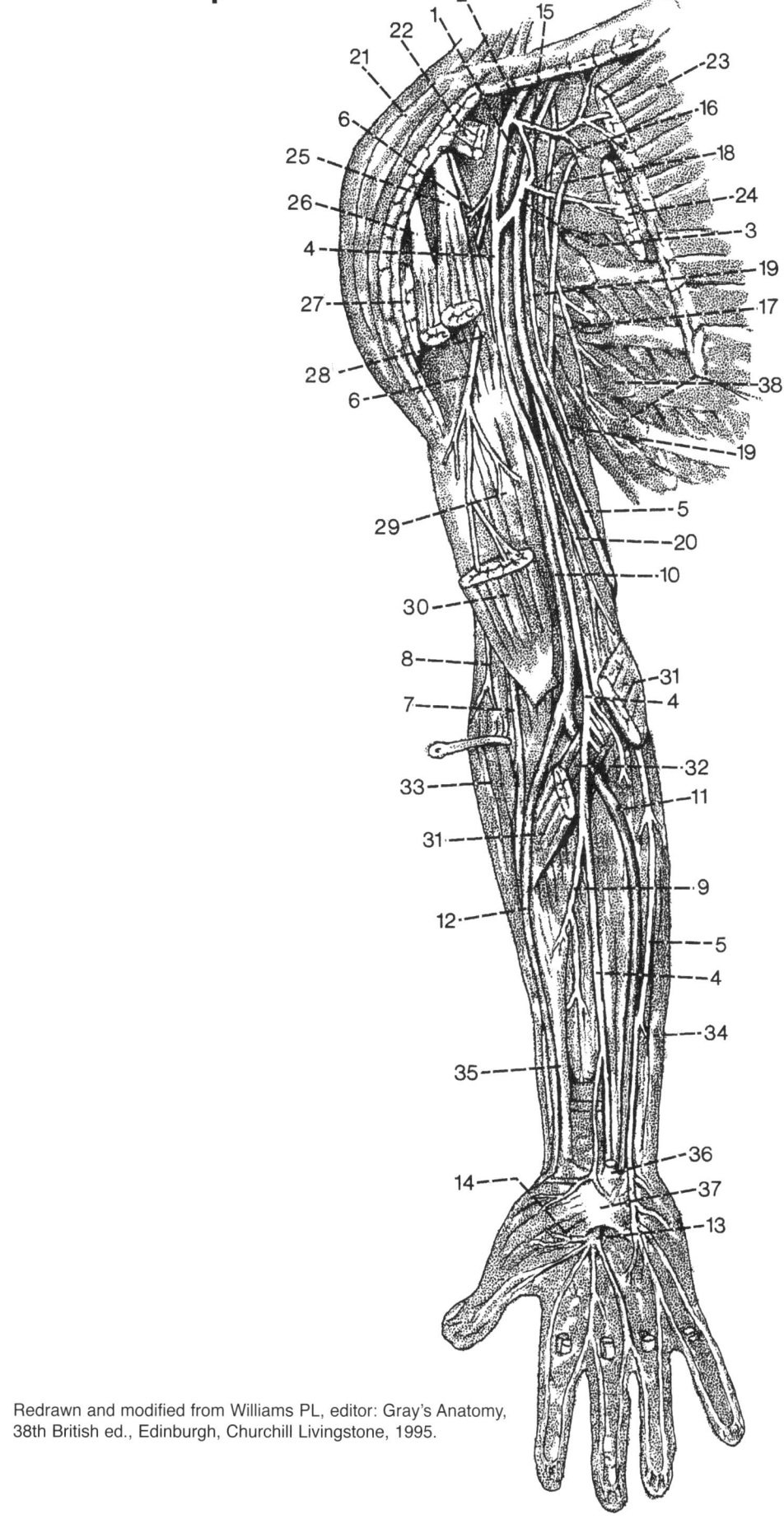

Redrawn and modified from Williams PL, editor: Gray's Anatomy, 38th British ed., Edinburgh, Churchill Livingstone, 1995.

23 Dissection of upper arm

Anterior aspect

Color and label

1. Median nerve
2. Axillary artery (it becomes brachial artery (7) at lower border of teres major)
3. Pectoralis major muscle (arm is abducted approximately 45° from the thorax)
4. Subscapularis muscle
5. Teres major muscle
6. Subscapular nerve (above) and subscapular artery (below)
7. Brachial artery
8. Ulnar nerve
9. Superior ulnar collateral artery
10. Medial intermuscular septum. This membranous partition separates the anterior flexor muscles from the posterior extensor triceps brachii, as does the lateral intermuscular septum (not shown). The ulnar nerve penetrates the medial intermuscular septum. The opening for the ulnar nerve has been removed.
11. Inferior ulnar collateral artery
12. Bicipital aponeurosis (old name, lacertus fibrosis)
13. Medial epicondyle of humerus
14. Pronator teres (humeral or superficial head)
15. Ulnar artery. After passing under the bicipital aponeurosis the brachial artery divides into the radial and ulnar arteries.
16. Flexor carpi ulnaris (humeral head)
17. Median nerve in forearm. Entering the forearm the median nerve passes under the bicipital aponeurosis and between the two heads of the pronator teres.
18. Cephalic vein
19. Deltoid muscle
20. Brachialis muscle
21. Biceps brachii muscle
22. Lower portion of brachialis muscle. This strong flexor of the forearm inserts on the ulnar tuberosity.
23. Tendon of biceps inserting on radial tuberosity
24. Brachial artery emerging from under the bicipital aponeurosis
25. Recurrent radial artery
26. Brachioradialis muscle
27. Superficial radial nerve
28. Radial artery

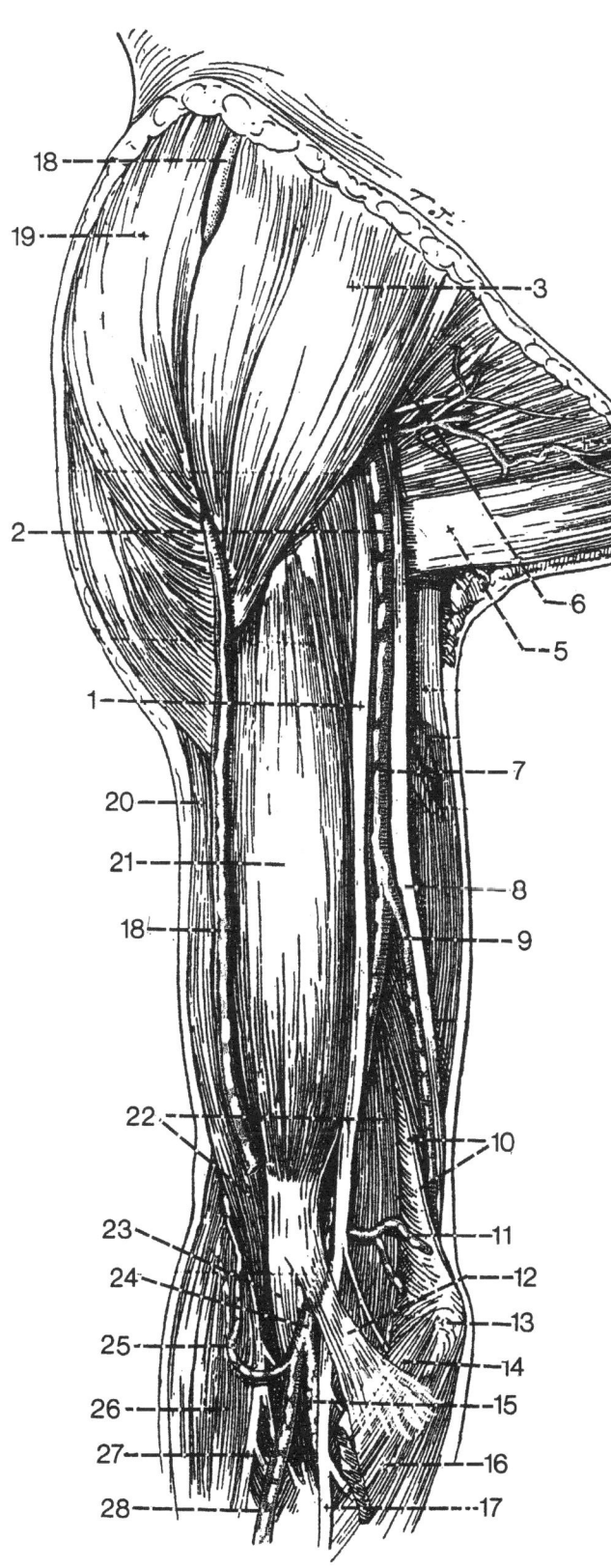

Eycleshymer and Jones with modification

24 Biceps brachii: a flexor and supinator

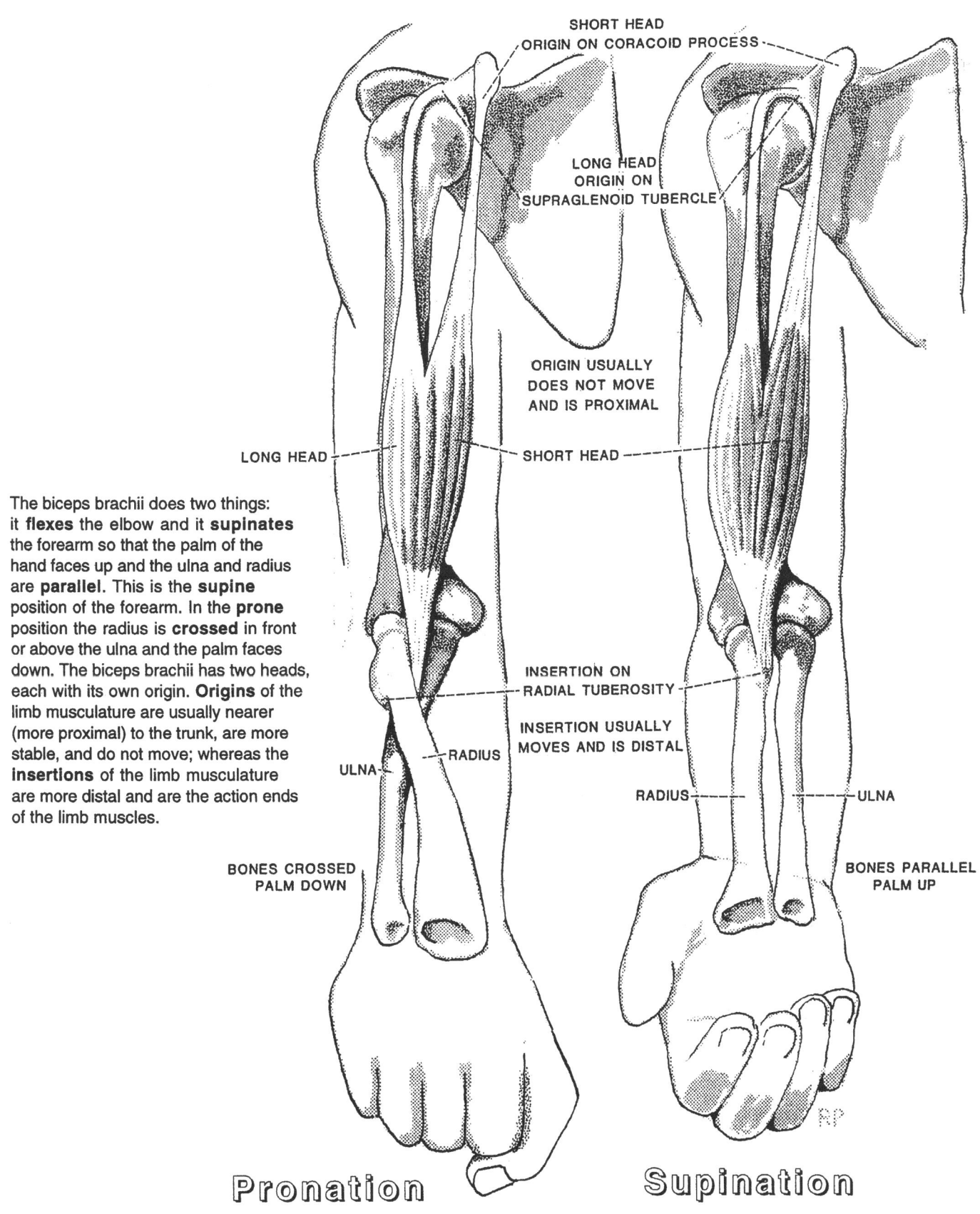

The biceps brachii does two things: it **flexes** the elbow and it **supinates** the forearm so that the palm of the hand faces up and the ulna and radius are **parallel**. This is the **supine** position of the forearm. In the **prone** position the radius is **crossed** in front or above the ulna and the palm faces down. The biceps brachii has two heads, each with its own origin. **Origins** of the limb musculature are usually nearer (more proximal) to the trunk, are more stable, and do not move; whereas the **insertions** of the limb musculature are more distal and are the action ends of the limb muscles.

25 Anterior forearm dissection

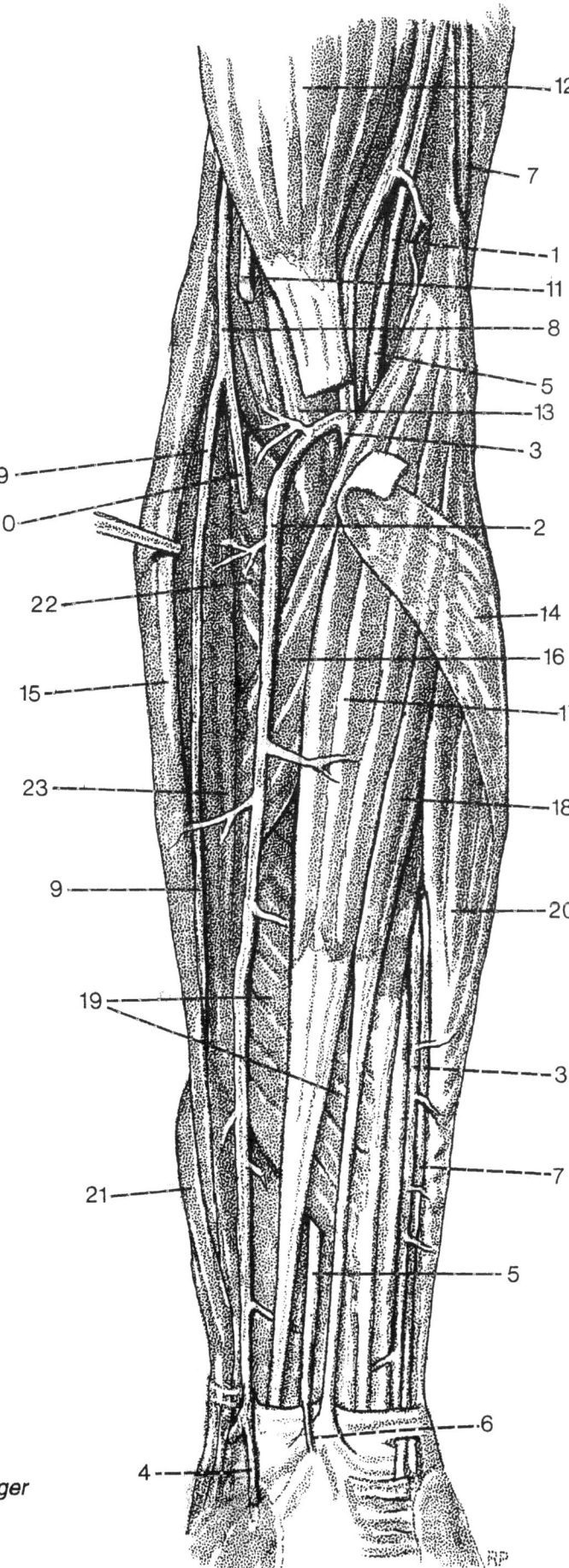

Color and label

1. Brachial artery
2. Radial artery
3. Ulnar artery
4. Superficial palmar branch of radial nerve
5. Median nerve (in upper arm and forearm)
6. Palmar branch of median nerve
7. Ulnar nerve
8. Radial nerve
9. Superficial branch of radial nerve
10. Deep branch of radial nerve
11. Musculocutaneous nerve (cut); becomes lateral cutaneous nerve of forearm
12. Biceps brachii muscle
13. Tendon of biceps brachii
14. Bicipital aponeurosis (cut)
15. Brachioradialis muscle
16. Pronator teres muscle
17. Flexor carpi radialis muscle
18. Palmaris longus muscle
19. Flexor digitorum superficialis
20. Flexor carpi ulnaris muscle
21. Abductor pollicis longus muscle
22. Supinator muscle
23. Extensor carpi radialis longus muscle

Redrawn from Wolf-Heidegger

26 Arteries and nerves of the anterior forearm

Color and label

1. Brachial artery
2. Ulnar artery
3. Radial artery
4. Ulnar recurrent artery
5. Common interosseous artery
6. Anterior interosseous artery
7. Posterior interosseous artery
8. Recurrent radial artery
9. Radial collateral artery
10. Inferior ulnar collateral artery
11. Superior ulnar collateral artery
12. Superficial palmar branch of ulnar artery
13. Deep palmar branch of ulnar artery
14. Superficial palmar branch of radial artery
15. Radial nerve
16. Median nerve
17. Anterior interosseous nerve; supplies deep flexor muscles of the forearm
18. Palmar branch of median nerve
19. Ulnar nerve
20. Superficial branch of median nerve
21. Deep branch of ulnar nerve
22. Lateral antebrachial cutaneous nerve (continuation of musculocutaneous nerve) (cut)
23. Deep branch of radial nerve
24. Superficial branch of radial nerve
25. Biceps brachii muscle
26. Tendon of biceps brachii
27. Bicipital aponeurosis (cut)
28. Common head of forearm flexors (cut)
29. Brachioradialis muscle (cut)
30. Flexor carpi ulnaris (cut)
31. Abductor pollicis longus muscle
32. Flexor pollicis longus muscle
33. Pronator quadratus muscle
34. Flexor digitorum profundus muscle; note that its four tendons remain flat as they pass into the hand
35. Four tendons of flexor digitorum superficialis (cut); note that tendons 3 and 4 to the middle and ring finger are anterior to tendons 2 and 5 which go to the index and little finger. Remember, when demonstrating with your own fingers and palm facing up: "34 is higher than 25".

Redrawn from Wolf-Heidegger

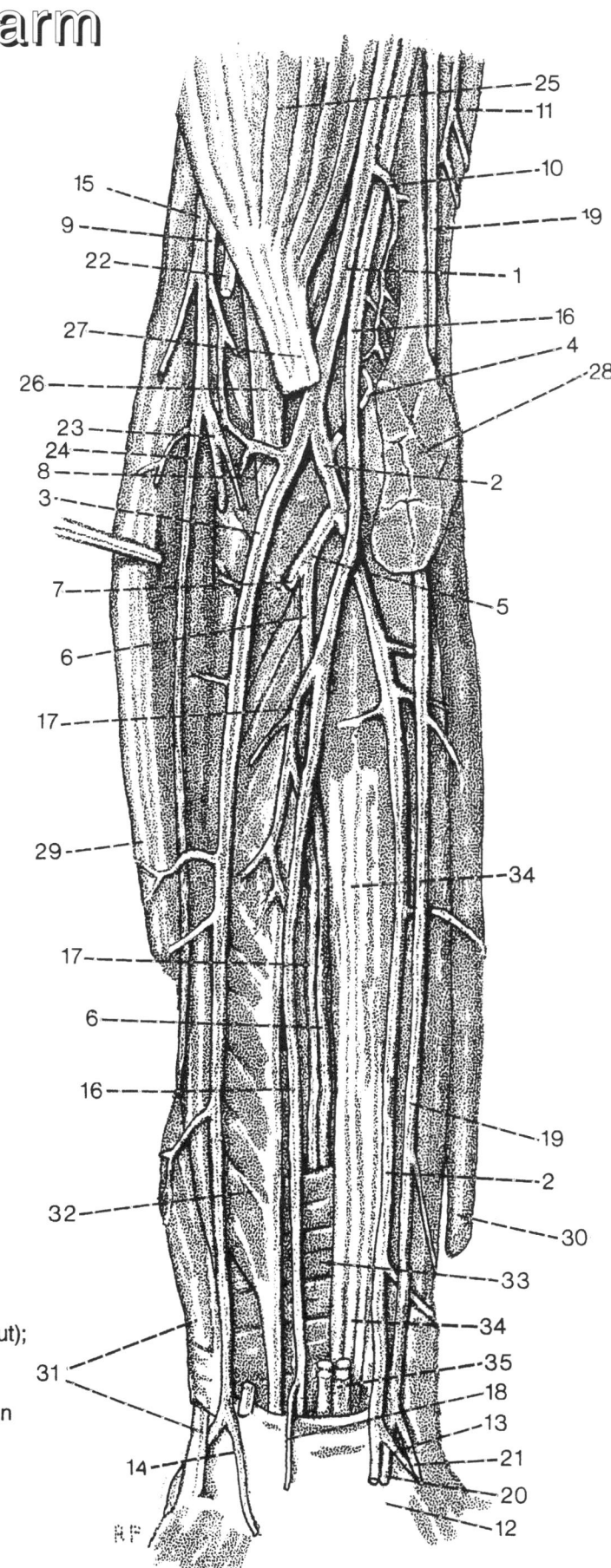

27 Brachial plexus and major nerves of the arm
Highly schematic

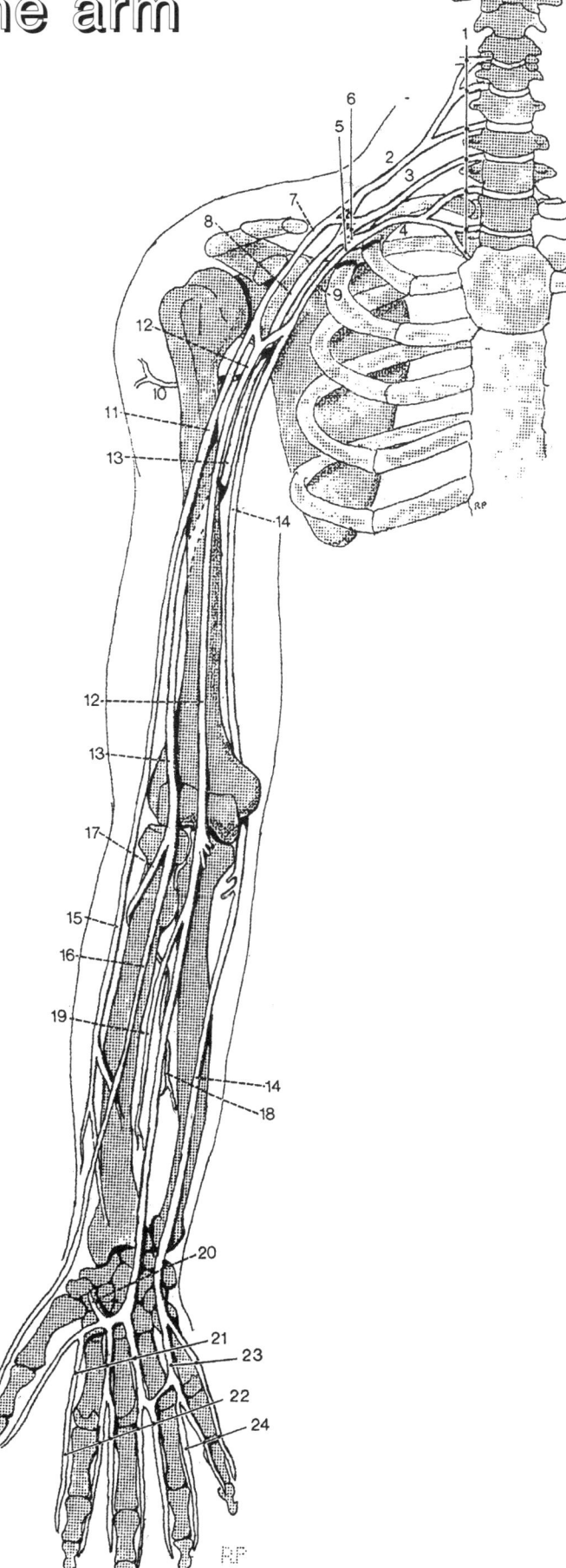

Color and label

1. Anterior rami of spinal nerves C4-T2 (small contributions from C4 and T2)
2. Superior trunk of brachial plexus
3. Middle trunk of brachial plexus
4. Inferior trunk of brachial plexus
5. Anterior divisions of three trunks
6. Posterior divisions of three trunks
7. Lateral cord
8. Posterior cord
9. Medial cord
10. Axillary nerve
11. Musculocutaneous nerve
12. Median nerve
13. Radial nerve
14. Ulnar nerve
15. Lateral cutaneous nerve of forearm (lateral antebrachial cutaneous nerve)
16. Superficial branch of radial nerve
17. Deep branch of radial nerve
18. Posterior interosseous nerve (continuation of deep branch of radial nerve)
19. Anterior interosseous nerve of median nerve
20. Thenar muscular branch of median nerve
21. Common palmar digital nerves (branches of median nerve)
22. Proper palmar digital nerves (of median nerve)
23. Common palmar digital nerves (branches of ulnar nerve)
24. Proper palmar digital nerves (of ulnar nerve)

Usually the skin of the fourth (ring) finger (or digit) is supplied by both the median nerve (laterally) and the ulnar nerve (medially).

28 Pronator teres and superficial wrist flexors (opposite page)

Color and label

1. Median nerve; supplies all the forearm wrist flexors except the flexor carpi ulnaris (ulnar nerve) and the two medial heads of the flexor digitorum profundus (ulnar nerve).
2. Pronator teres muscle (humeral or superficial head)
3. Pronator teres muscle (ulnar or deep head); both heads supplied by median nerve.
4. Flexor carpi radialis muscle (median nerve)
5. Palmaris longus muscle (median nerve)
6. Palmar aponeurosis; a strong triangular portion of deep fascia in the palm of the hand. It receives the tendon of the palmaris longus.
7. Flexor carpi unlnaris muscle (ulnar nerve)
8. Pisiform (pea-shaped) bone. One of the carpal bones. The flexor carpi ulnaris inserts on it.
9. Flexor retinaculum. It forms the roof of the carpal tunnel through which run the flexor tendons of the fingers and the median nerve.
10. Brachioradialis (radial nerve)
11. Extensor carpi radialis longus (radial nerve)

Muscles are described in terms of their Origin, Insertion, Action, Innervation

Muscle	Origin	Insertion	Action	Innervation
Flexor carpi radialis	Medial epicondyle of humerus by common flexor tendon, and the antebrachial fascia and the intermuscular fascia	Base of second metacarpal plus a slip to the third metacarpal	Flexes and abdusts the hand	Median nerve
Palmaris longus	Common flexor tendon (medial humeral epicondyle) and antebrachial fascia	Flexor retinaculum and palmar aponeurosis	Flexes the hand and tenses the palmar aponeurosis	Median nerve
Brachioradialis	Upper two thirds of the supracondylar ridge of the humerus and the front of the lateral intermuscular septum	Base of styloid process of radius	Flexes forearm, especially in the semiprone position, and helps in pronation when the arm is supine and flexed	Branch of radial nerve with fibers from nerves C5 and C6
Flexor carpi ulnaris humeral head	Common flexor tendon (medial humeral epicondyle)	Pisiform bone and by the pisohamate and pisometacarpal ligaments to the hamate bone and the base of the fifth metacarpal bone	Helps flex and adduct the hand	Ulnar nerve
Flexor carpi ulnaris ulnar head	Medial side of the olecranon and upper two thirds of the posterior margin of the ulna			

28 Pronator teres and superficial wrist flexors

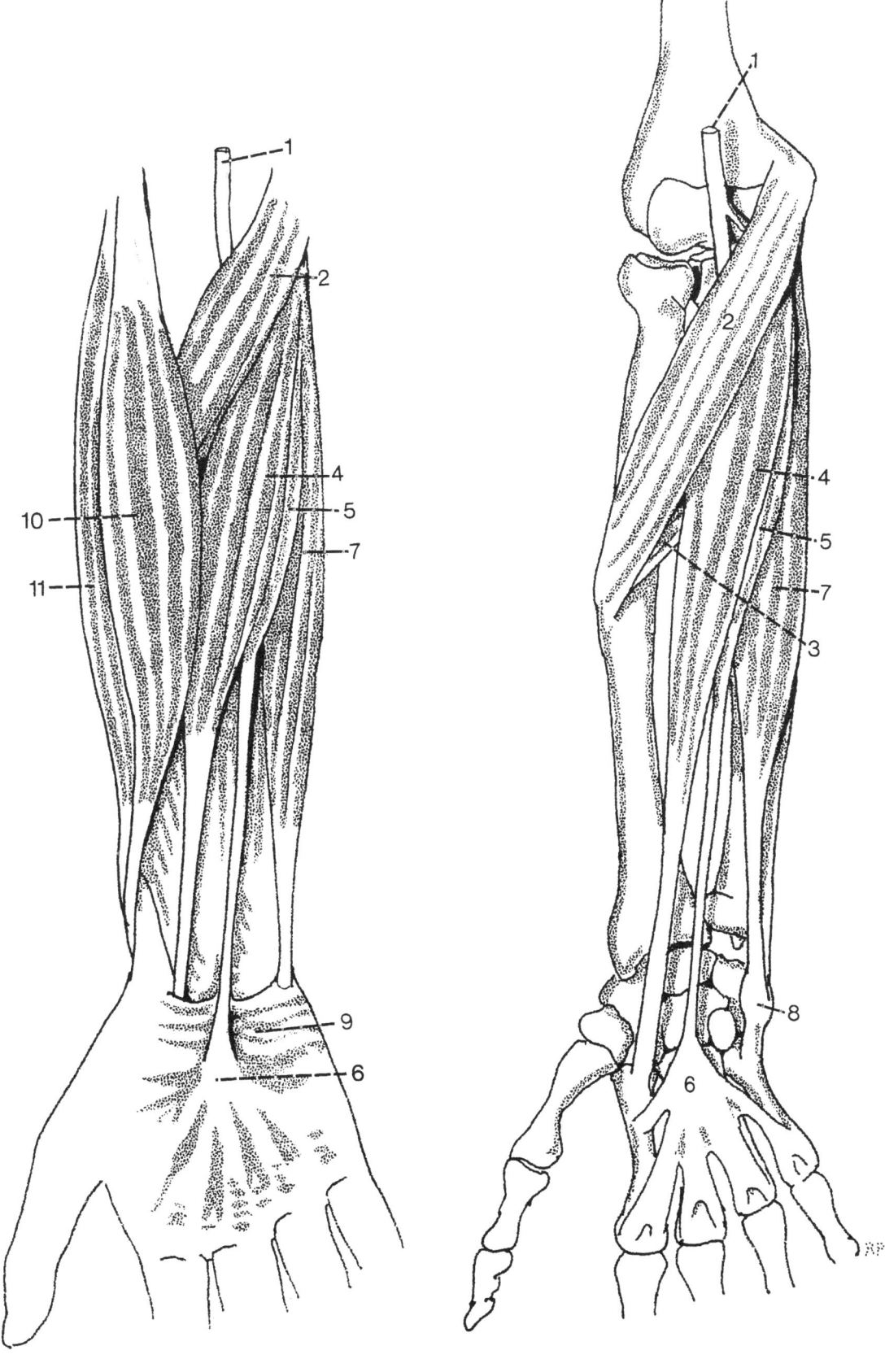

29 Musculocutaneous nerve and the muscles it supplies

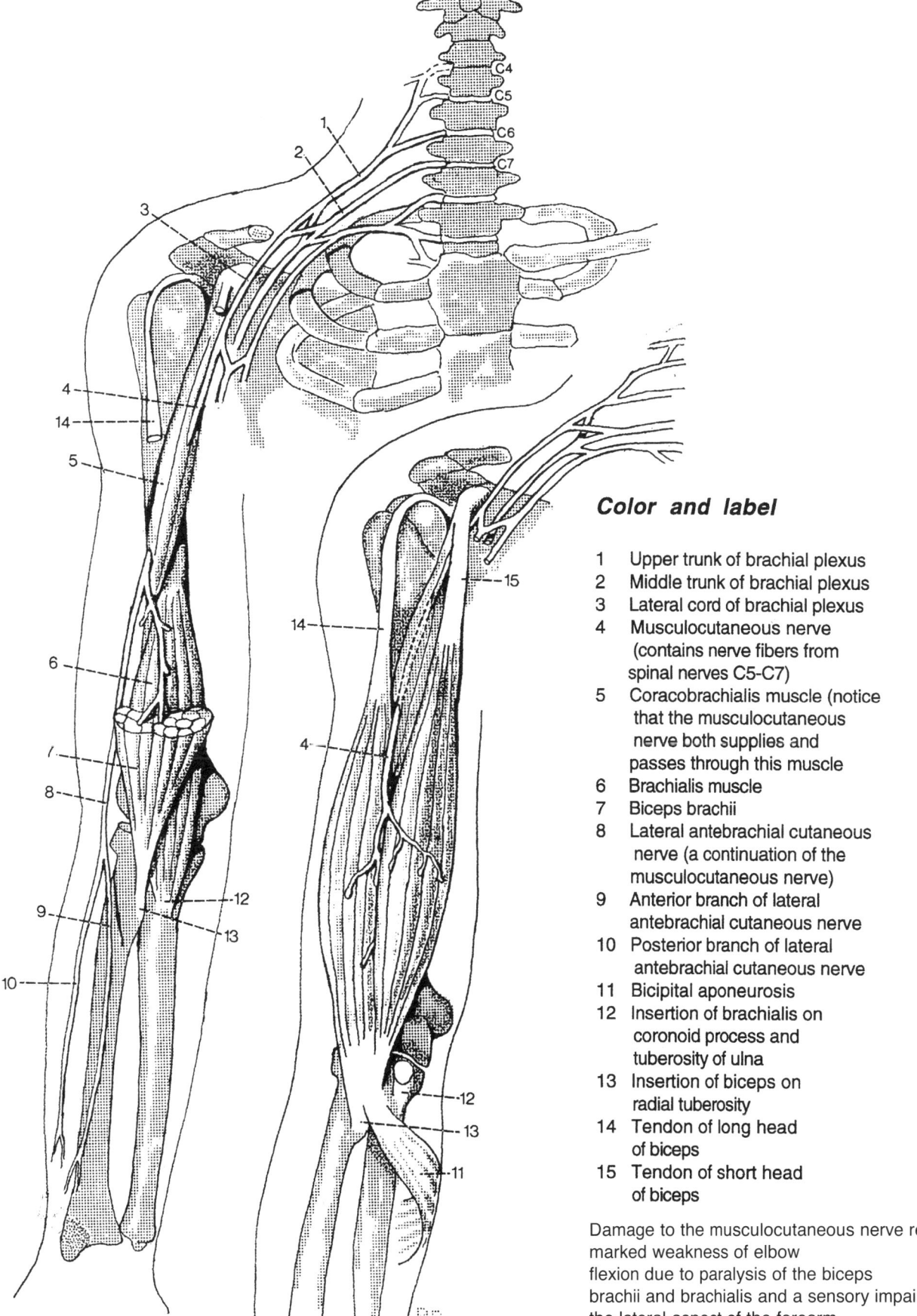

Color and label

1. Upper trunk of brachial plexus
2. Middle trunk of brachial plexus
3. Lateral cord of brachial plexus
4. Musculocutaneous nerve (contains nerve fibers from spinal nerves C5-C7)
5. Coracobrachialis muscle (notice that the musculocutaneous nerve both supplies and passes through this muscle)
6. Brachialis muscle
7. Biceps brachii
8. Lateral antebrachial cutaneous nerve (a continuation of the musculocutaneous nerve)
9. Anterior branch of lateral antebrachial cutaneous nerve
10. Posterior branch of lateral antebrachial cutaneous nerve
11. Bicipital aponeurosis
12. Insertion of brachialis on coronoid process and tuberosity of ulna
13. Insertion of biceps on radial tuberosity
14. Tendon of long head of biceps
15. Tendon of short head of biceps

Damage to the musculocutaneous nerve results in marked weakness of elbow flexion due to paralysis of the biceps brachii and brachialis and a sensory impairment to the lateral aspect of the forearm.

30 Muscular distribution of the median nerve

Damage to the median nerve high in the forearm may result in weakness in pronation, weakness in the long finger flexors (weak grip), and sensory impairment on the palm of the hand. The most common entrapment of median nerve is the **carpal tunnel syndrome** caused by compression of the median nerve as it passes through the carpal tunnel into the hand under the flexor retinaculum. Various factors may cause the carpal tunnel to become narrowed, resulting in wasting and weakness of the abductor pollicis brevis and impairment of sensation in the thumb, index and middle fingers, and lateral side of the ring finger.

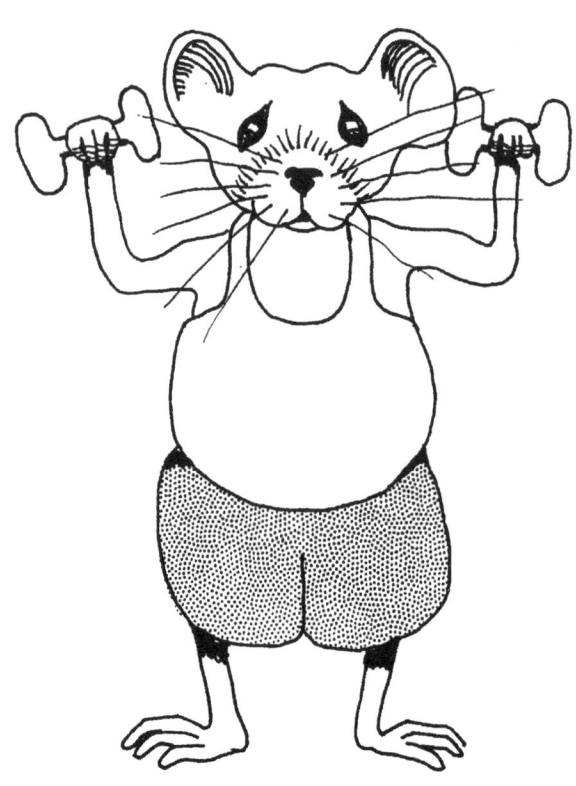

Muscle means "Little Mouse"

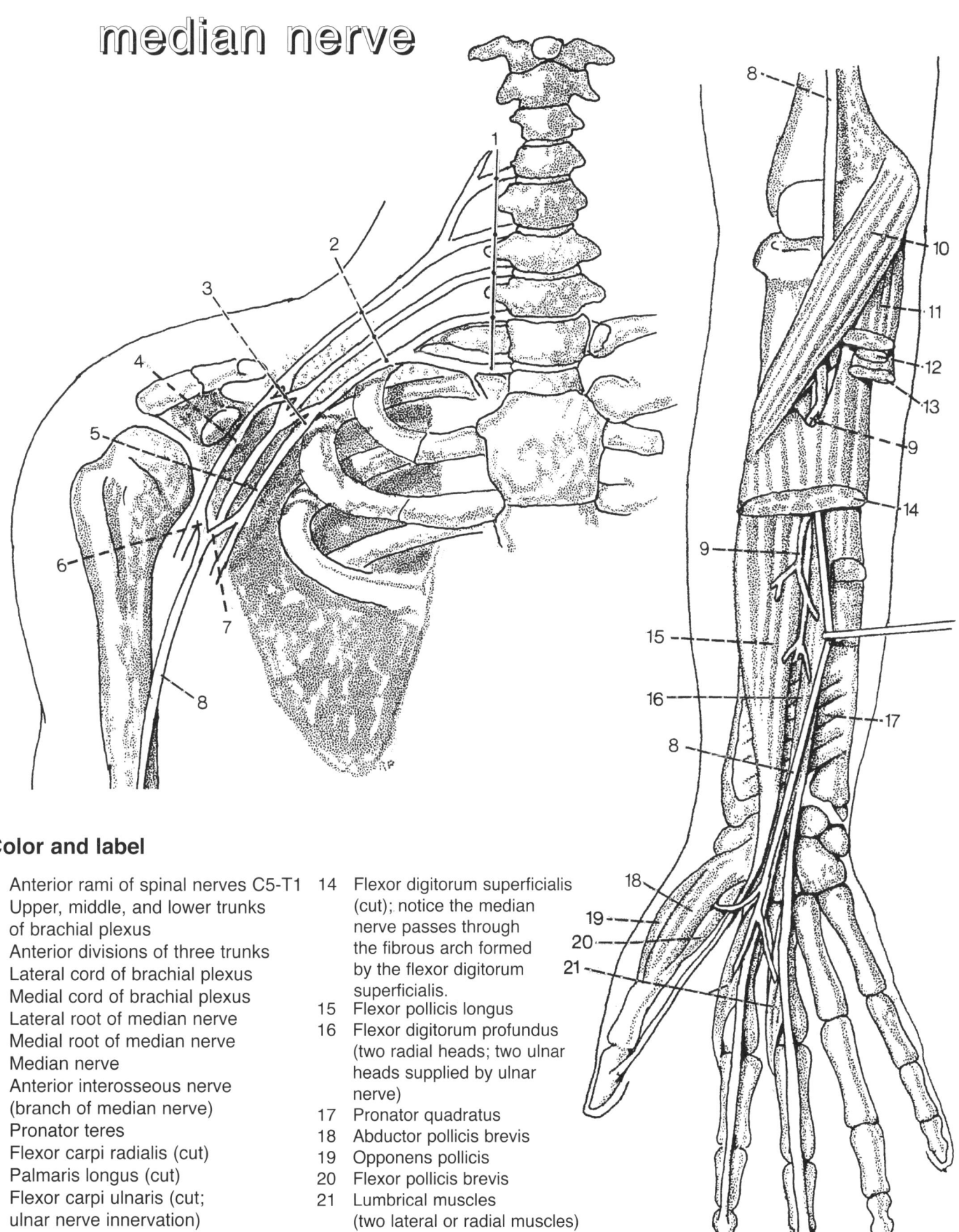

30 Muscular distribution of the median nerve

Color and label

1. Anterior rami of spinal nerves C5-T1
2. Upper, middle, and lower trunks of brachial plexus
3. Anterior divisions of three trunks
4. Lateral cord of brachial plexus
5. Medial cord of brachial plexus
6. Lateral root of median nerve
7. Medial root of median nerve
8. Median nerve
9. Anterior interosseous nerve (branch of median nerve)
10. Pronator teres
11. Flexor carpi radialis (cut)
12. Palmaris longus (cut)
13. Flexor carpi ulnaris (cut; ulnar nerve innervation)
14. Flexor digitorum superficialis (cut); notice the median nerve passes through the fibrous arch formed by the flexor digitorum superficialis.
15. Flexor pollicis longus
16. Flexor digitorum profundus (two radial heads; two ulnar heads supplied by ulnar nerve)
17. Pronator quadratus
18. Abductor pollicis brevis
19. Opponens pollicis
20. Flexor pollicis brevis
21. Lumbrical muscles (two lateral or radial muscles)

31 Flexor digitorum superficialis muscle

Color and label

1. Flexor digitorum superficialis; notice that as its four tendons pass through the concavity of the carpal tunnel they become "squeezed" so that the tendons to fingers 3 and 4 become anterior to the tendons to fingers 2 and 5. A helpful mnemonic: "34 is higher than 25" (with the palm facing up)
2. Flexor digitorum superficialis tendon(s); notice how the superficial flexor tendons end by dividing on the proximal phalanx of the four medial fingers to allow passage through them of the corresponding tendon of the flexor digitorum profundus; they then reunite, decussate (6), divide again, and insert on the sides of the middle phalanx (7).
3. Flexor digitorum profundus tendon (cut)
4. Short vinculum* (pl. vincula)
5. Long vinculum**
6. Decussation of the tendon of the flexor digitorum superficialis
7. Insertion of its tendon on sides of middle phalanx

*(Vinculum, Latin, a band). The short vincula are short triangular tendinous folds that attach the finger flexor tendons to the interphangeal joints and adjacent parts of the phalanges. There are two short vincula in each finger; the proximal short vinculum attaches the superficial flexor tendon near its insertion to the proximal interphangeal joint; the distal short vinculum attaches the deep (profundus) flexor tendon to the distal interphangeal joint and adjacent bones.

** There are three long vincula in each finger. The proximal long vincula are two slender threadlike bands connecting each side of the superficial flexor tendon to the synovial sheath at the lateral border near the base of the proximal phalanx. The single distal long vinculum connects the tendon of the profundus flexor to the posterior part of the synovial sheath at the distal end of the proximal phalanx.

31 Flexor digitorum superficialis muscle

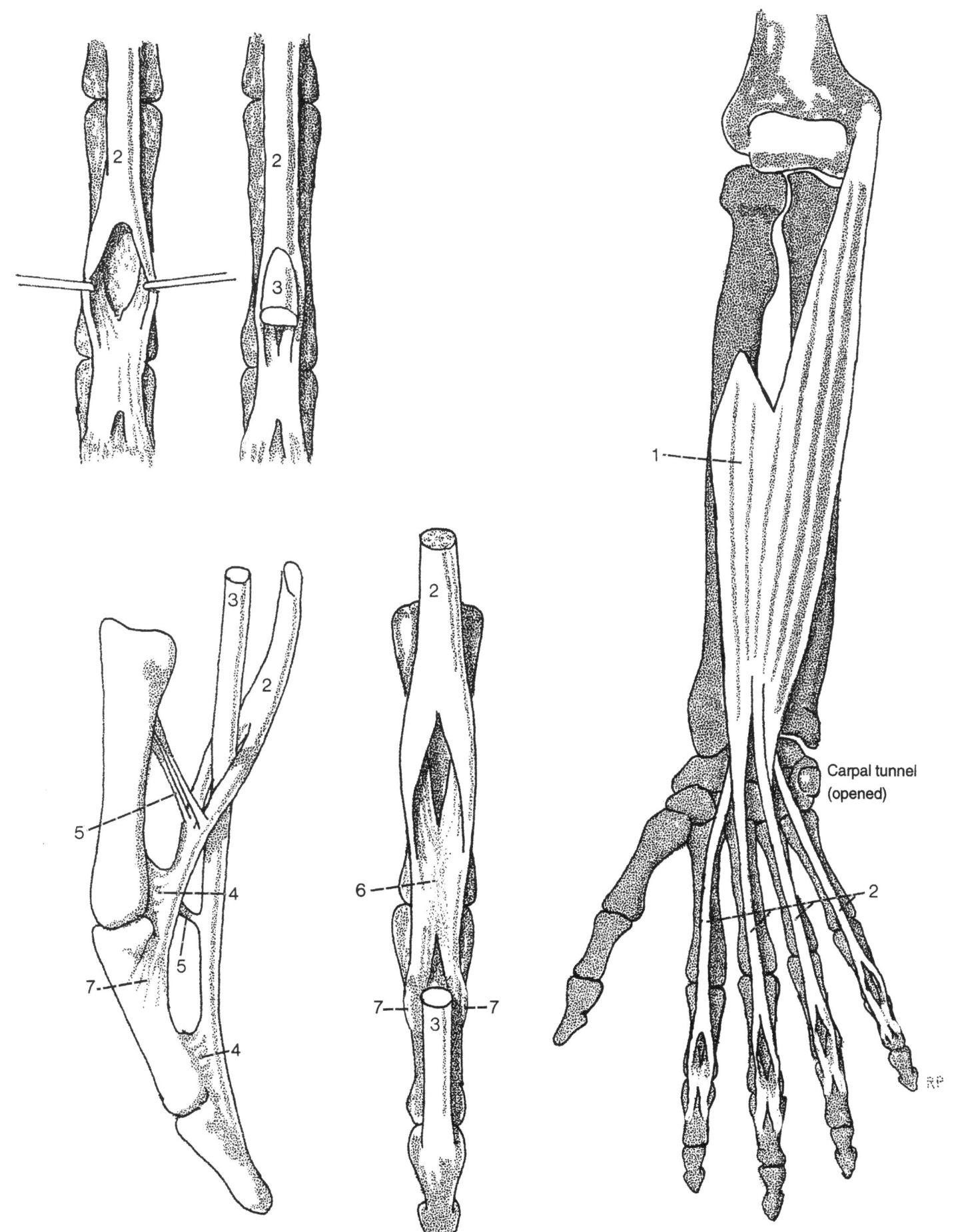

32 Flexor pollicis longus, flexor digitorum profundus, and median nerve

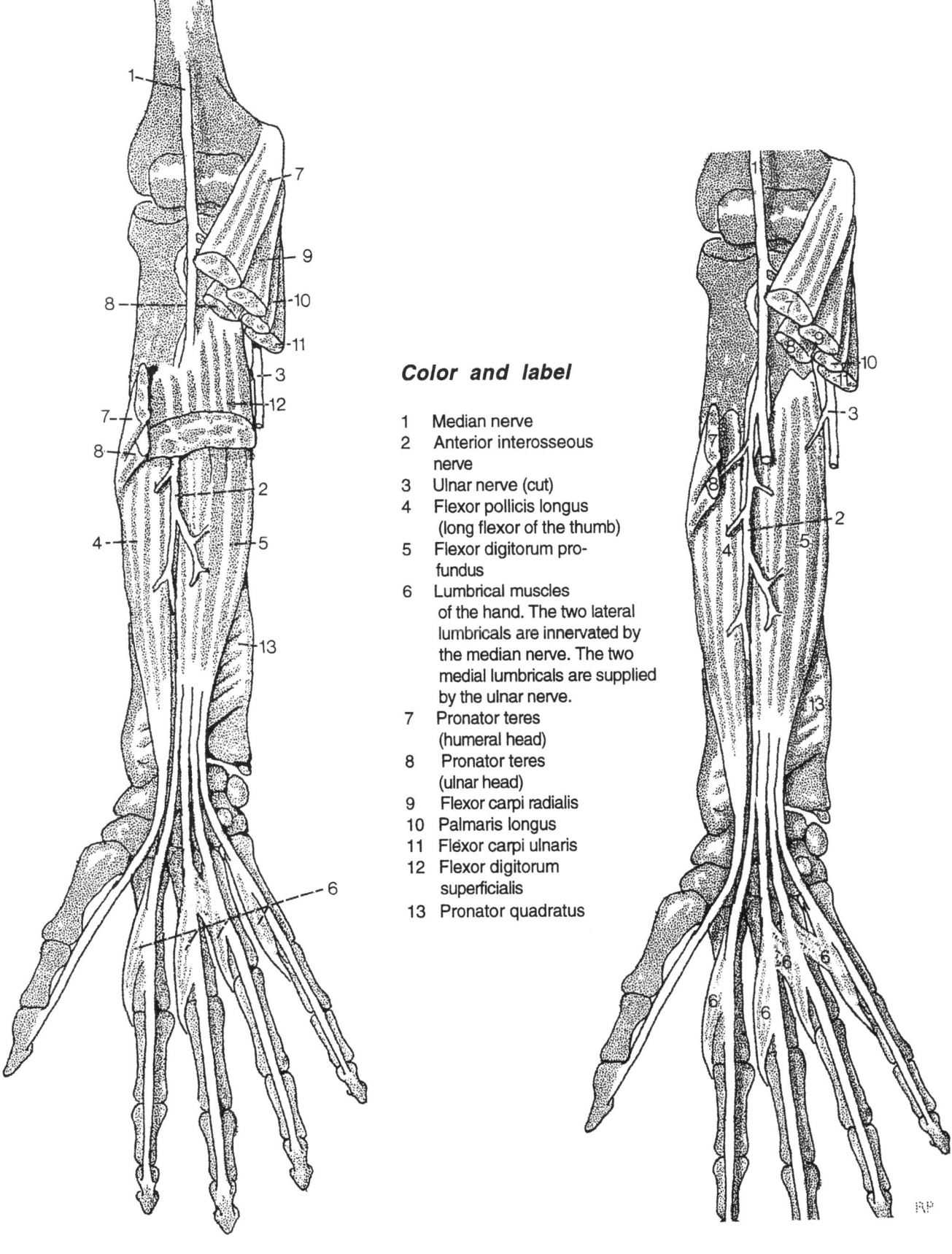

Color and label

1. Median nerve
2. Anterior interosseous nerve
3. Ulnar nerve (cut)
4. Flexor pollicis longus (long flexor of the thumb)
5. Flexor digitorum profundus
6. Lumbrical muscles of the hand. The two lateral lumbricals are innervated by the median nerve. The two medial lumbricals are supplied by the ulnar nerve.
7. Pronator teres (humeral head)
8. Pronator teres (ulnar head)
9. Flexor carpi radialis
10. Palmaris longus
11. Flexor carpi ulnaris
12. Flexor digitorum superficialis
13. Pronator quadratus

33 Median nerve and deep dissection of the forearm

Color and label

1. Median nerve
2. Anterior antebrachial interosseous nerve (also anterior interosseous nerve of the forearm). It supplies the flexor pollicis longus, flexor digitorum profundus (two lateral heads), and the pronator quadratus, plus sensory receptors on the interosseous membrane and distally the radioulnar, radiocarpal, and carpal joints.
3. Ulnar nerve
4. Flexor pollicis longus muscle
5. Flexor digitorum profundus muscle
6. Lumbrical muscles of the fingers. Notice how the four lumbrical muscles arise from the four tendons of the deep finger flexor; only the two lateral (radial) lumbricals are supplied by the median nerve (figure on right). The two medial lumbricals (ulnar nerve innervation) arise from two adjacent profundus tendons rather than from a single profundus tendon.
7. Pronator teres (humeral head)
8. Pronator teres (ulnar head)
9. Flexor carpi radialis muscle
10. Palmaris longus muscle
11. Flexor carpi ulnaris muscle
12. Flexor digitorum superficialis muscle
13. Pronator quadratus muscle
14. Opponens pollicis muscle
15. Abductor pollicis brevis muscle
16. Flexor pollicis brevis muscle
17. Motor branch of median nerve to thenar muscles
18. Common digital nerves
19. Proper digital nerves

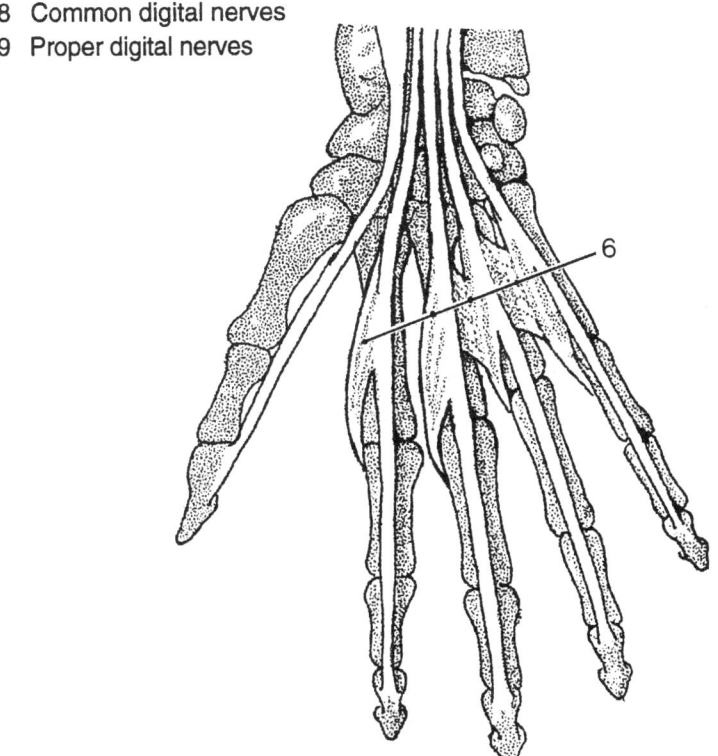

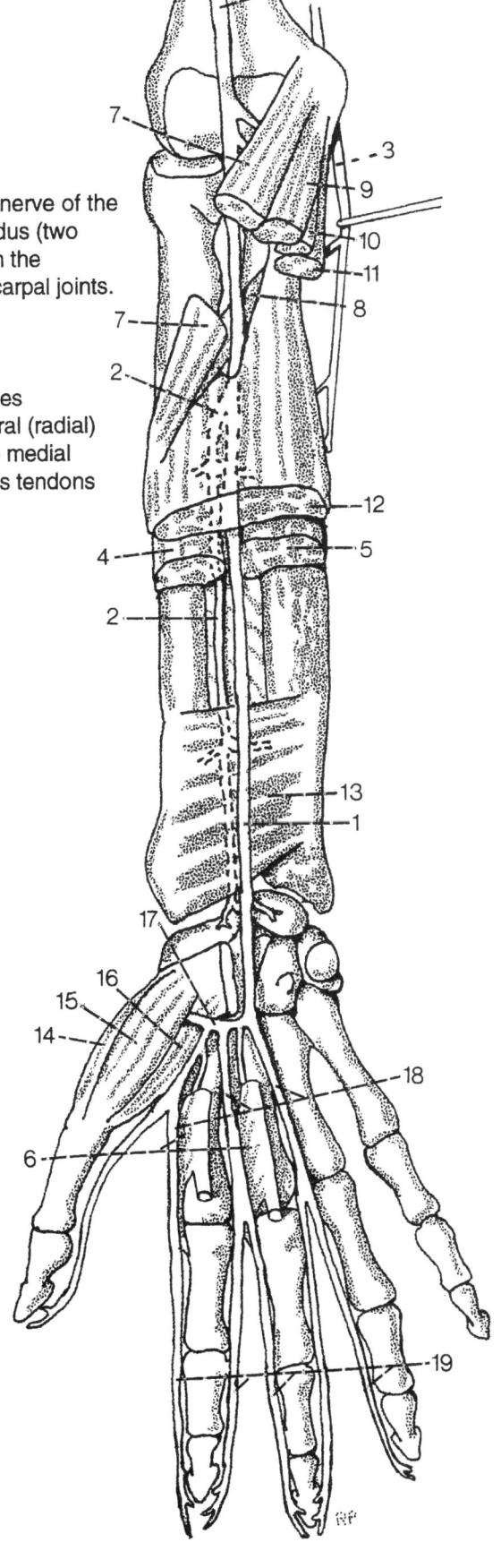

34 Motor distribution of the ulnar nerve

Color and label

1. Upper trunk of brachial plexus
2. Middle trunk of brachial plexus
3. Lower trunk of brachial plexus
4. Medial cord of brachial plexus
5. Posterior cord of brachial plexus
6. Lateral cord of brachial plexus
7. Ulnar nerve (the continuation of the medial cord with fibers mainly from C8 and T1)
8. Median nerve
9. Musculocutaneous nerve
10. Radial nerve
11. Axillary nerve
12. Medial intermuscular septum

Muscles innervated by ulnar nerve

13. Flexor carpi ulnaris
14. Flexor digitorum profundus (two medial heads)
15. Abductor digiti minimi
16. Flexor digiti minimi
17. Medial two lumbricals
18. Adductor pollicis (transverse and oblique heads)
19. Palmar interosseous muscles (bring fingers together; adduct)
20. Dorsal interosseous muscles (spread apart fingers; abduct)
21. Deep branch of ulnar nerve
22. Superficial branch of ulnar nerve

Also supplied by ulnar nerve
opponens digiti minimi
deep head of flexor pollicis brevis
palmaris brevis

* Ulnar nerve penetrating medial intermuscular septum

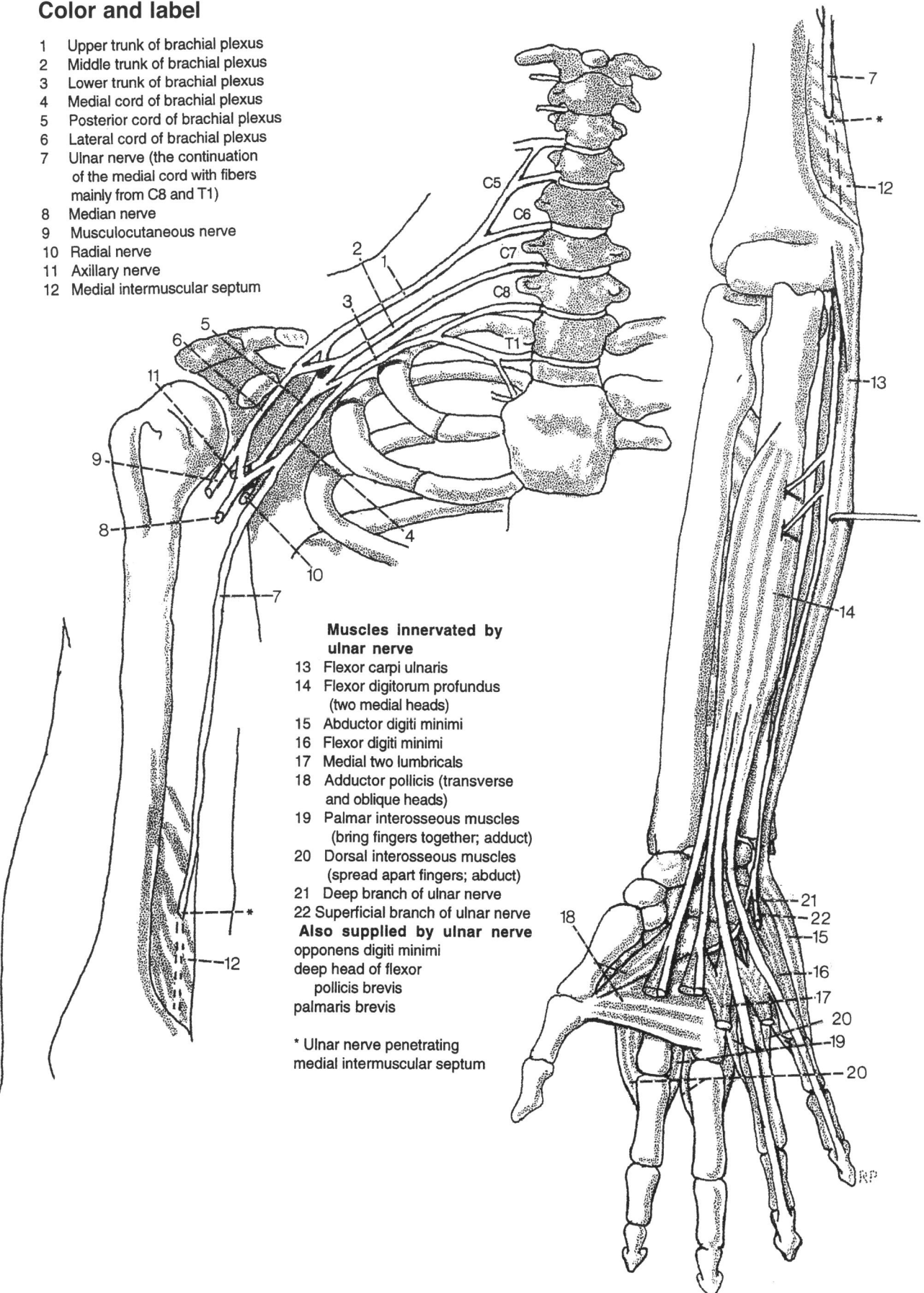

35 Motor distribution of the radial nerve I

Superficial muscles

The radial nerve is the largest nerve in the arm. The radial nerve and the axillary nerve both arise from the posterior cord of the brachial plexus. Because it spirals downward directly on the humerus, the radial nerve may be injured in fractures of the humerus. The radial nerve innervates all the extensors of the elbow, wrist, and fingers. It does not, however, supply any intrinsic hand musculature.

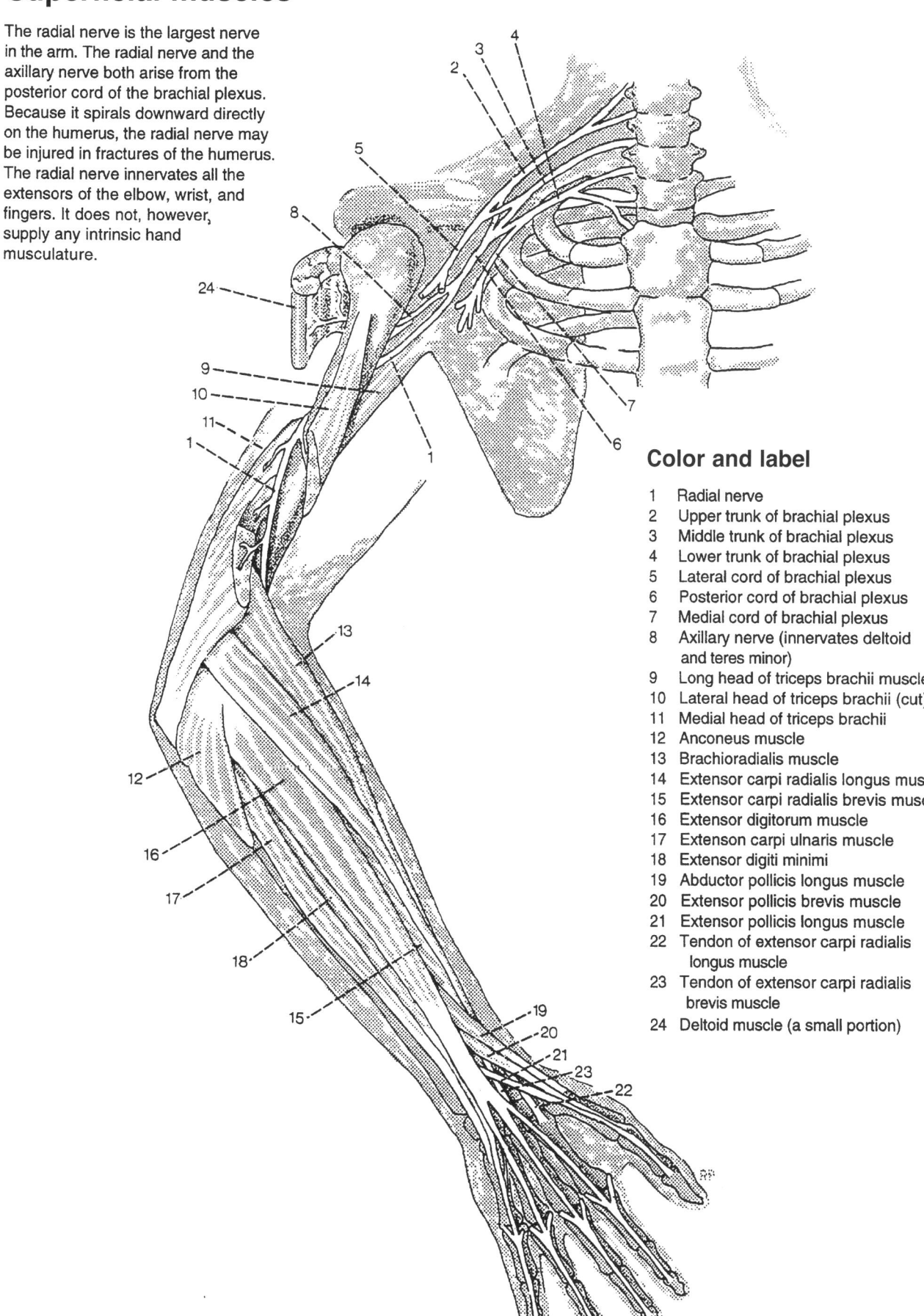

Color and label

1. Radial nerve
2. Upper trunk of brachial plexus
3. Middle trunk of brachial plexus
4. Lower trunk of brachial plexus
5. Lateral cord of brachial plexus
6. Posterior cord of brachial plexus
7. Medial cord of brachial plexus
8. Axillary nerve (innervates deltoid and teres minor)
9. Long head of triceps brachii muscle
10. Lateral head of triceps brachii (cut)
11. Medial head of triceps brachii
12. Anconeus muscle
13. Brachioradialis muscle
14. Extensor carpi radialis longus muscle
15. Extensor carpi radialis brevis muscle
16. Extensor digitorum muscle
17. Extenson carpi ulnaris muscle
18. Extensor digiti minimi
19. Abductor pollicis longus muscle
20. Extensor pollicis brevis muscle
21. Extensor pollicis longus muscle
22. Tendon of extensor carpi radialis longus muscle
23. Tendon of extensor carpi radialis brevis muscle
24. Deltoid muscle (a small portion)

36 Motor distribution of radial nerve II
Deep muscles

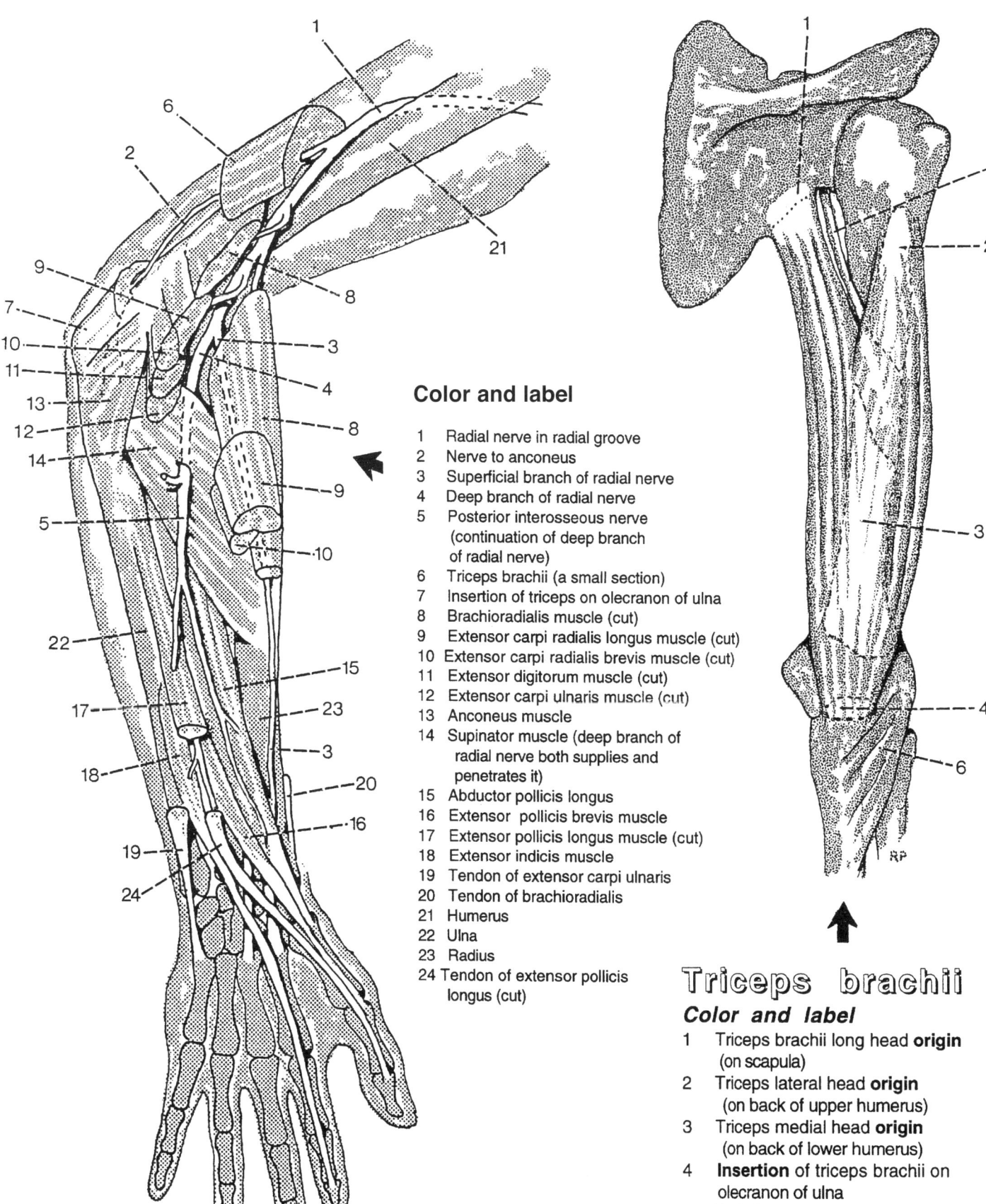

Color and label

1. Radial nerve in radial groove
2. Nerve to anconeus
3. Superficial branch of radial nerve
4. Deep branch of radial nerve
5. Posterior interosseous nerve (continuation of deep branch of radial nerve)
6. Triceps brachii (a small section)
7. Insertion of triceps on olecranon of ulna
8. Brachioradialis muscle (cut)
9. Extensor carpi radialis longus muscle (cut)
10. Extensor carpi radialis brevis muscle (cut)
11. Extensor digitorum muscle (cut)
12. Extensor carpi ulnaris muscle (cut)
13. Anconeus muscle
14. Supinator muscle (deep branch of radial nerve both supplies and penetrates it)
15. Abductor pollicis longus
16. Extensor pollicis brevis muscle
17. Extensor pollicis longus muscle (cut)
18. Extensor indicis muscle
19. Tendon of extensor carpi ulnaris
20. Tendon of brachioradialis
21. Humerus
22. Ulna
23. Radius
24. Tendon of extensor pollicis longus (cut)

Triceps brachii
Color and label

1. Triceps brachii long head **origin** (on scapula)
2. Triceps lateral head **origin** (on back of upper humerus)
3. Triceps medial head **origin** (on back of lower humerus)
4. **Insertion** of triceps brachii on olecranon of ulna
5. Radial nerve
6. Anconeus muscle

37 Bones of the hand
(opposite page)

Palmar (ventral) aspect of right hand

Color and label

1. Scaphoid (boat-shaped; old name, navicular)
2. Lunate (moon-shaped)
3. Triquetral (three-cornered)
4. Pisiform (resembling a pea)
5. Trapezium (resembling a Greek small table called a *trapezion;* old name, greater multangular)
6. Trapezoid (resembling a quadrilateral figure which has two parallel sides; old name, lesser multangular)
7. Capitate (having a head or an enlargement)
8. Hamate (hook-shaped; *hamus*, Latin, a hook)
9. First metacarpal (of thumb); the five metacarpal bones are the largest and strongest bones in the hand.
10. Base of fifth metacarpal
11. Body of fifth metacarpal
12. Head of fifth metacarpal (each metacarpal bone has a base, body, and head)
13. Base of proximal phalanx of index finger
14. Body of proximal phalanx of index finger
15. Head of proximal phalanx of index finger
16. Middle phalanx of index finger
17. Distal phalanx of index finger (each phalanx has a base, body, and head)
18. Proximal phalanx of thumb
19. Distal phalanx of thumb; the thumb, which is the most mobile and useful finger, has only two phalanges, whereas each of the other four digits has three phalanges, resulting in 14 phalanges in each hand.
20. Radial sesamoid bone (resembling a sesame seed)
21. Ulnar sesamoid bone (sesamoid bones develop within tendons and remain in them)
22. Tuberosity of distal phalanx
23. Hamulus (Latin, little hook) of hamate bone
24. Tubercle of trapezium
25. Tubercle of scaphoid
26. Carpometacarpal joint; the thumb carpometacarpal joint is a saddle joint.
27. Metacarpophalangeal joint (abbreviated MP joint or MCP joint)
28. Proximal interphalangeal joint (PIP joint)
29. Distal interphalangeal joint (DIP joint)

37 Bones of the hand

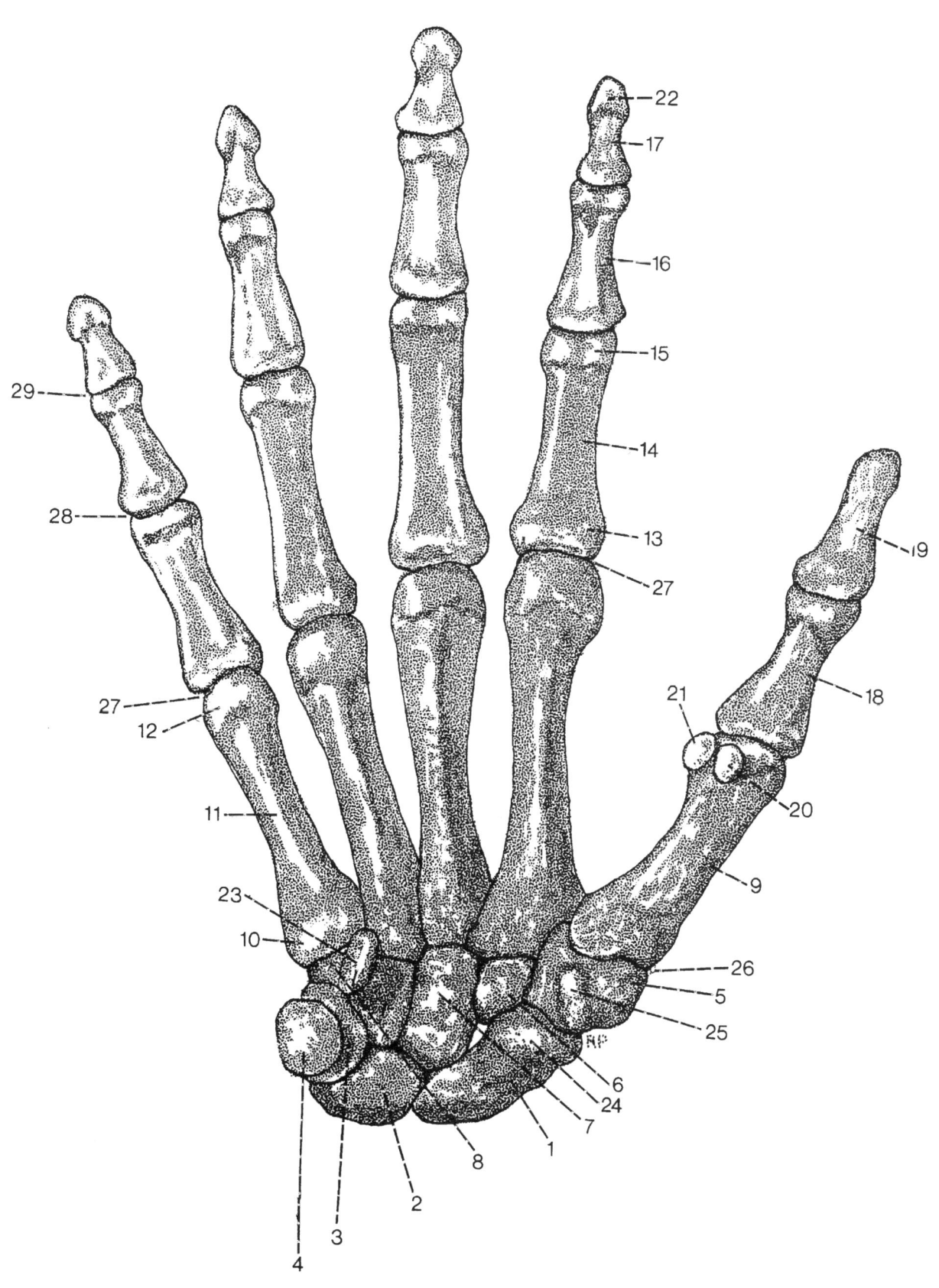

Phalanx
(etymological cartoon)

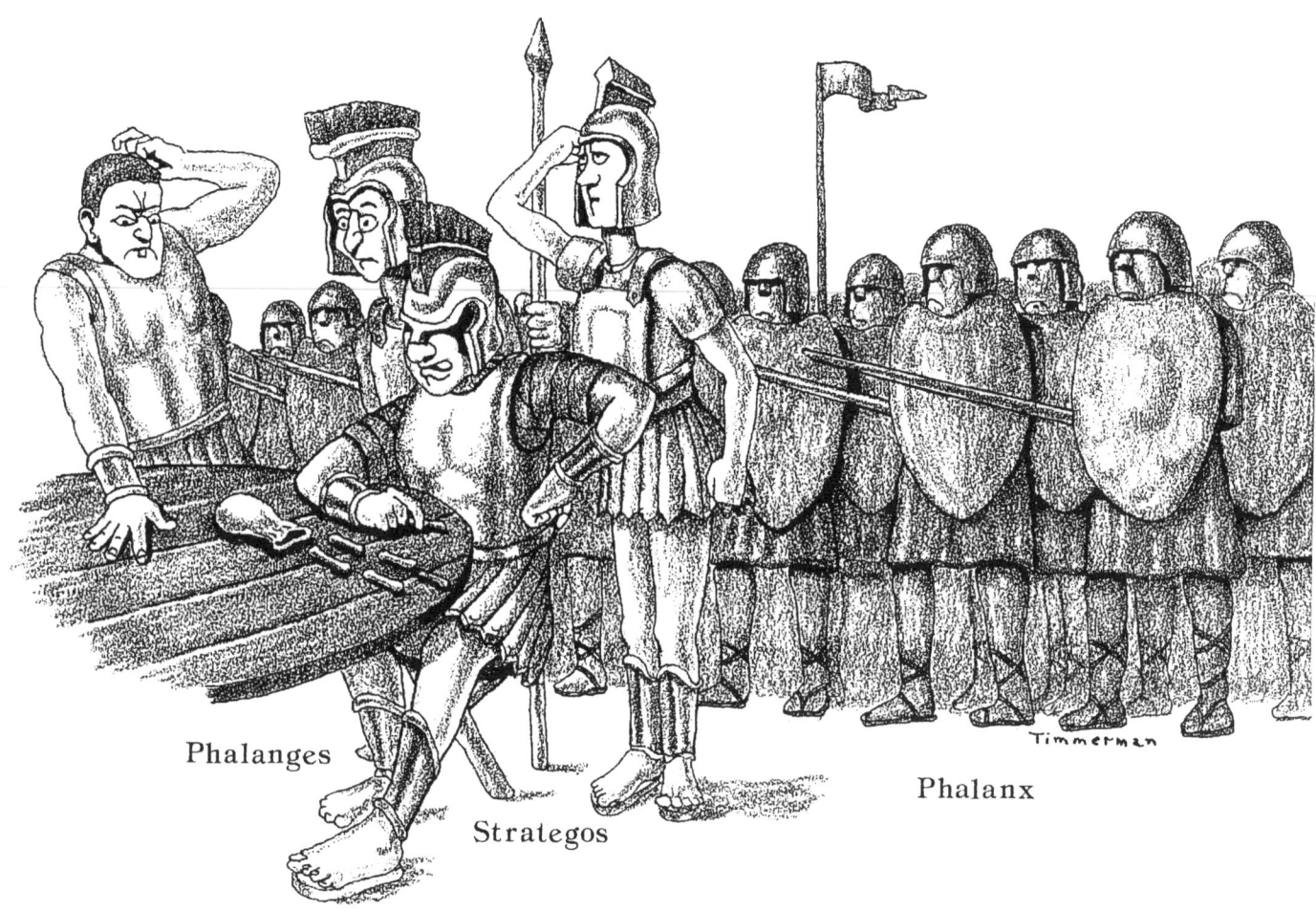

Phalanges
Strategos
Phalanx

Phalanx

Phalanx (Greek) was a compact formation of infantry soldiers with overlapping shields and projecting spears. It was developed by Philip II of Macedon and later used extensively by Alexander the Great.

The ***phalanges*** (plural of *phalanx*) are the bones of the fingers and toes. Supposedly it was Aristotle who gave them this name. He thought that the bones within the fingers resembled a formation of infantry phalanges drawn up for battle. The thumb (*pollex*, Latin) has only two phalanges as does the big toe (*hallux*, Latin). The rest of the fingers (digits 2-5) each has three phalanges; thus each hand and each foot has fourteen phalanges (2+3+3+3+3=14). The wrist (*carpus*, Latin) consists of eight carpal bones in two rows of four. Within the palm of the hand are the five metacarpal (beyond the carpus) bones. These are the largest and strongest bones of the hand, especially the second and third metacarpal bones which directly receive the force of impact when the fist strikes a blow. The foot has seven tarsal bones, five metatarsal bones, and fourteen phalanges. *Tarsos* was Greek for a flat surface, or sole of the foot, or edge of the eyelid. In anatomy the tarsus refers specifically to the instep of the foot or to that part of the foot containing the seven tarsal bones.

A Greek general was a ***strategos***, hence our word *strategy*. Army was *stratos* and "to lead" was *agein*, thus to be a general or "to lead an army" was *stratos* + *agein* = *strategein* which got shortened to *strategos*.

38 Palmar aponeurosis and anchoring connective tissue

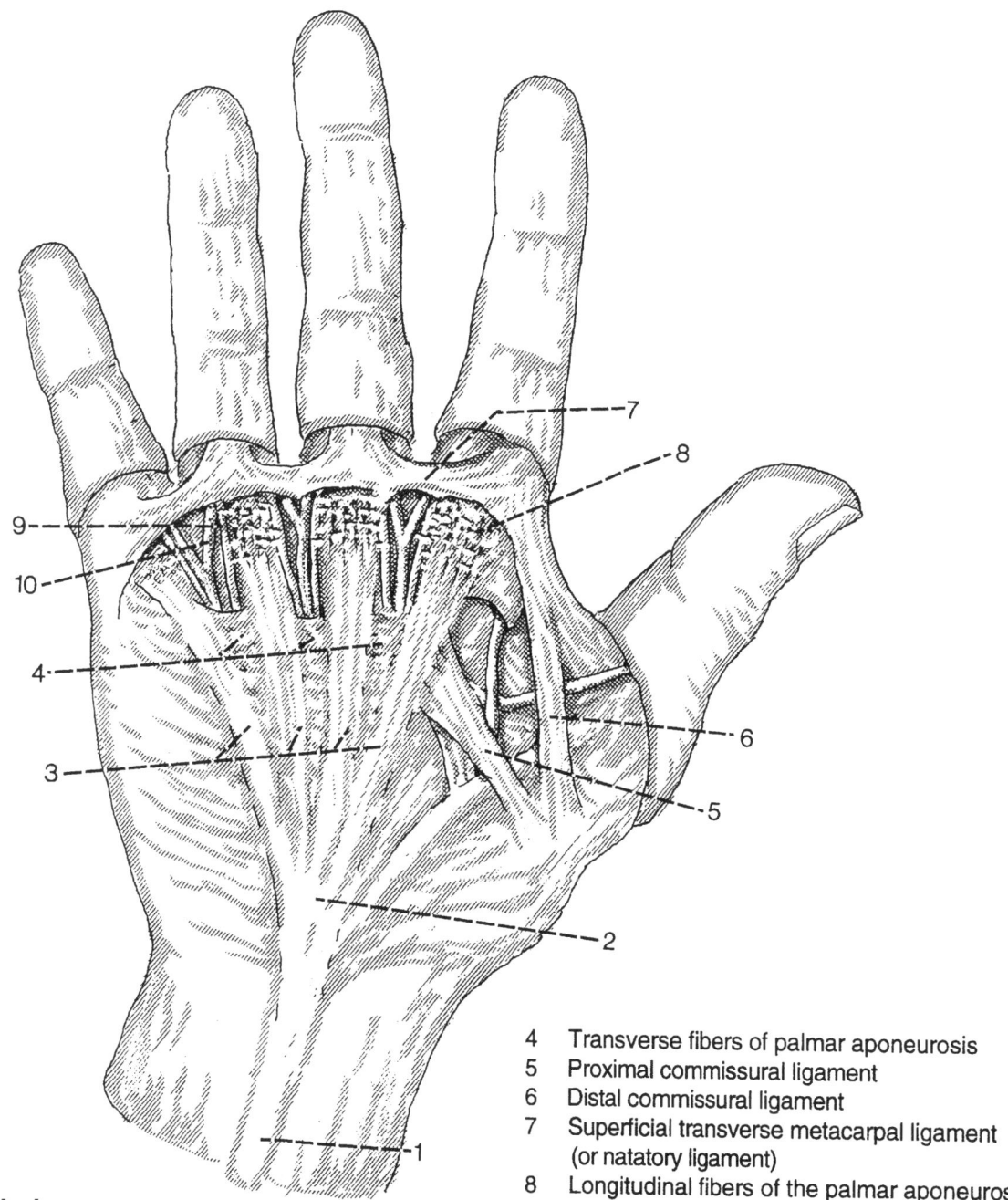

4 Transverse fibers of palmar aponeurosis
5 Proximal commissural ligament
6 Distal commissural ligament
7 Superficial transverse metacarpal ligament (or natatory ligament)
8 Longitudinal fibers of the palmar aponeurosis inserting into the skin of the palm (cut when skin is removed). These superficial longitudinal fibers insert into the dermis of the distal palm, thus anchoring the skin of the palm and resisting centrifugal pulling or degloving forces that occur in, e.g., swinging a baseball bat.
9 Digital nerve (proper digital nerve)
10 Digital artery (proper digital artery)

Color and label

1 Tendon of palmaris longus muscle. When present this muscle by way of its long tendon inserts into the apex of the palmar aponeurosis.
2 Palmar aponeurosis. The thick triangular sheet of deep fascia in the palm of the hand. It is firmly bound to the overlying skin by its superficial fibers. Its deeper fibers join the fibrous flexor sheaths of the fingers.
3 Longitudinal fibers of palmar aponeurosis

Redrawn and modified from Williams PL: Gray's Anatomy, 38th British ed., Edinburgh, Churchill Livingstone, 1995.

39 Flexor retinaculum and superficial hand muscles
(opposite page)

After removal of palmar aponeurosis

Color and label

1. Flexor retinaculum; strong fibrous band in front of the wrist. It is continous with the antebrachial fascia. It forms the roof of the carpal tunnel by spanning the hollowed space formed by the carpal bones.
2. Tendons of flexor digitorum superficialis to digits 2-5
3. Tendon of flexor carpi radialis
4. Tendon of flexor pollicis longus
5. Tendon of abductor pollicis longus
6. Tendon of flexor carpi ulnaris
7. Pisiform bone (one of the eight carpal or wrist bones); the tendon of flexor carpi ulnaris inserts on it.
8. Abductor pollicis brevis (a thenar muscle)
9. Flexor pollicis brevis (a thenar muscle)
10. Opponens pollicis (a thenar muscle); these three very important muscles form the thenar eminence.
11. Adductor pollicis
12. Lumbrical muscles to digits 2-5; they arise from the radial side of the four tendons of flexor digitorum profundus which lie directly deep to the four flexor superficialis tendons.
13. First dorsal interosseous
14. Flexor digiti minimi
15. Abductor digiti minimi
16. Opponens digiti minimi; these three muscles (14, 15, 16) form the hypothenar eminence.
17. Cruciate (or crossing) fibers of fibrous tendon sheath; cruciate fibers occur at the interphalangeal joints and allow the sheaths to fold at the joints as the fingers flex.
18. Fibrous and synovial tendon sheaths of middle finger (opened)
19. Tendon of flexor digitorum profundus of middle finger; note its insertion on the distal phalanx.
20. Arrow in carpal tunnel
21. Annular fibers of fibrous tendon sheath. These are stronger and thicker than the cruciate fibers and hold the flexor tendons firmly against the phalanges, thus preventing them from bowing.

Redrawn from Wolf-Heidegger

39 Flexor retinaculum and superficial hand muscles

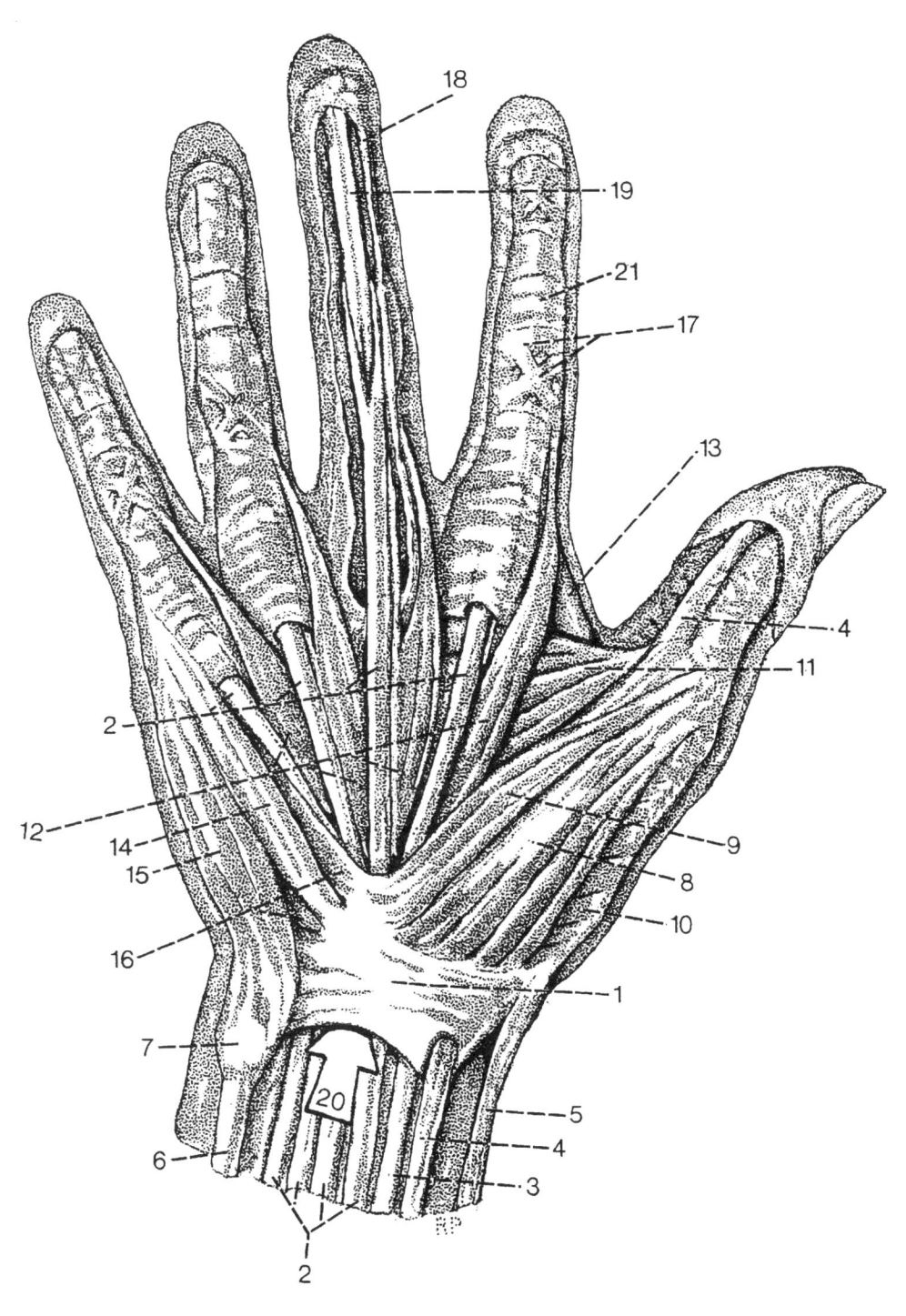

40 Deep thenar, hypothenar, and interosseous muscles

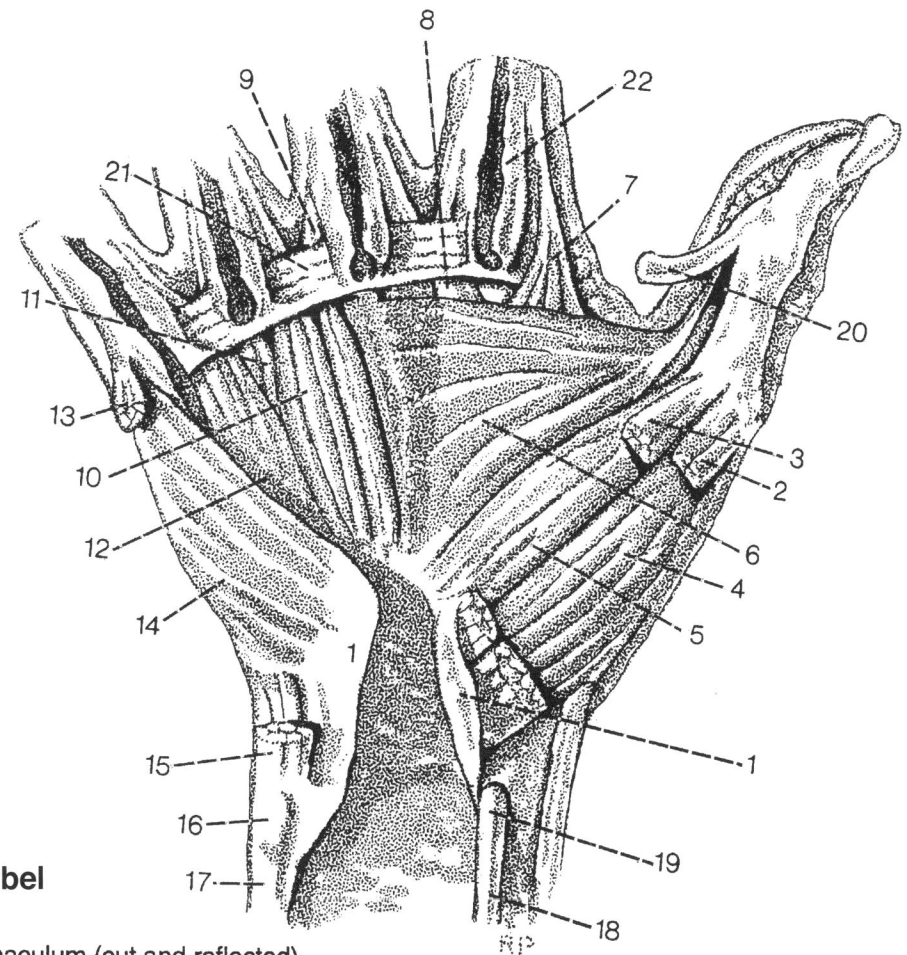

Color and label

1. Flexor retinaculum (cut and reflected)
2. Abductor pollicis brevis (cut). Supplied by the median nerve. It abducts the thumb, rotating it medially; flexes the proximal phalanx; and extends the terminal phalanx. (Also called short abductor muscle of the thumb)
3. Flexor pollicis brevis (cut); (superficial head). Supplied by recurrent branch of median nerve. (Also called short flexor muscle of the thumb)
4. Opponens pollicis. Supplied by the median nerve, it flexes, abducts, and medially rotates the first metacarpal in opposition. (Also called opposing muscle of the thumb)
5. Flexor pollicis brevis; (deep head). The deep head is usually supplied by the deep branch of the ulnar nerve.
6. Adductor pollicis. It arises by two heads: an oblique head (caput obliquum) and a transverse head (caput transversum). It is supplied by the deep branch of the ulnar nerve. It adducts and flexes the first metacarpal bone of the thumb, and flexes the proximal metacarpal of the thumb, especially in gripping movements.
7. First dorsal interosseous
8. First palmar interosseous
9. Third dorsal interosseous
10. Second palmar interosseous
11. Fourth dorsal interosseous
12. Third palmar interosseous
13. Common insertion of abductor digiti minimi and flexor digiti minimi (cut)
14. Opponens digiti minimi
15. Abductor digiti minimi (origin)
16. Pisiform bone
17. Tendon of flexor carpi ulnaris
18. Tendon of flexor carpi radialis
19. Tendon of abductor pollicis longus
20. Tendon of flexor pollicis longus
21. Deep transverse carpal ligament
22. Fibrous tendon sheath (cut open and both superficial and deep tendons removed)

Redrawn from Wolf-Heidegger

41 Interosseous and related muscles

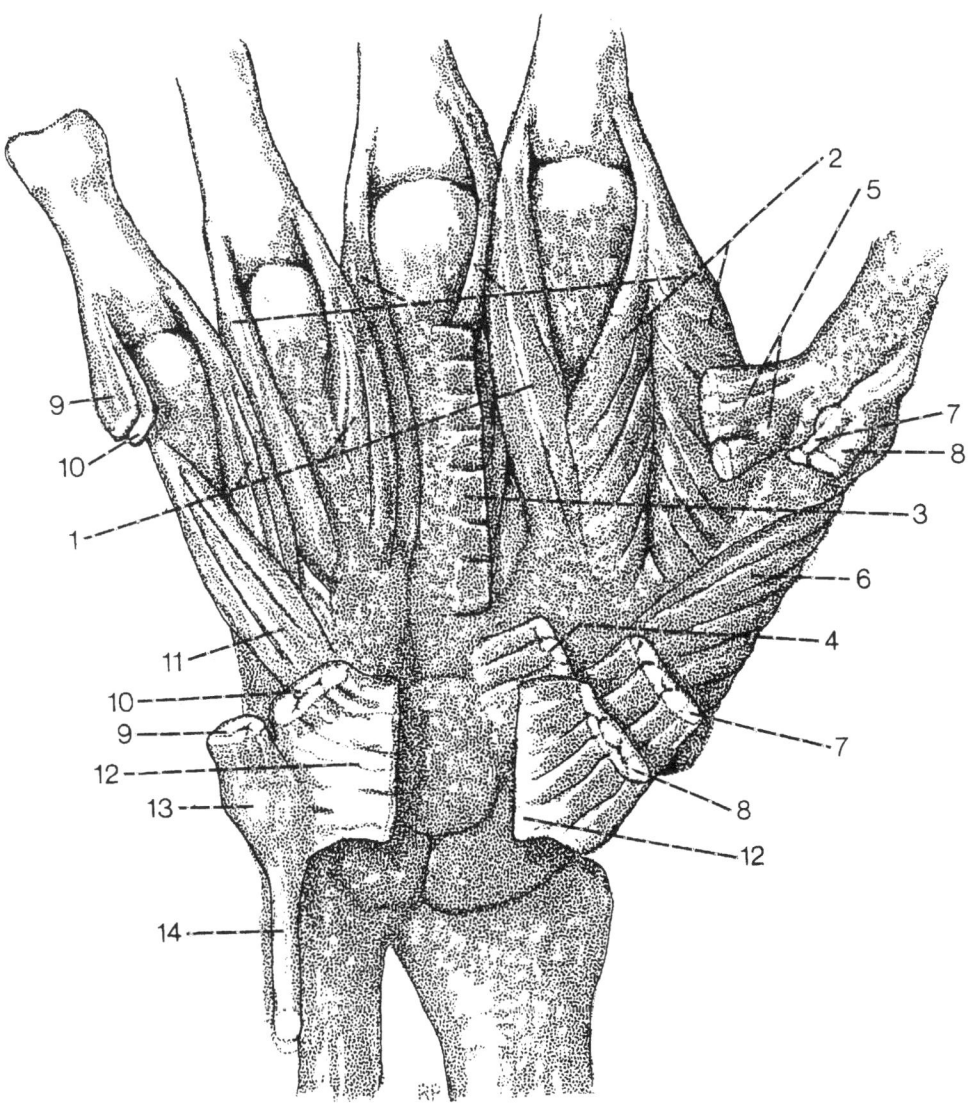

Color and label

1 Palmar interosseous muscles. The traditional view is that there are three of these muscles (as depicted here). However, some authors find that there are actually four, and that the first has been mistakenly overlooked as part of either the flexor pollicis brevis or the adductor pollicis. The palmar interossei adduct (bring together) digits 2, 4, and 5 toward the middle finger. They also flex the MP joint (metacarpophalangeal) and extend the PIP joint (proximal interphalangeal) and the DIP (distal interphalangeal) joint. They are supplied by the deep branch of the ulnar nerve.

2 Dorsal interosseous muscles. Four bipennate* muscles. They are supplied by the ulnar nerve. They abduct the second and fourth finger from the middle finger which itself remains stationary. Like the palmar interossei they flex the first phalanges and extend the middle and distal phalanges.

3 Adductor pollicis (transverse head, cut)
4 Adductor pollicis (oblique head, cut)
5 Adductor pollicis insertion with ulnar sesamoid bone
6 Opponens pollicis
7 Flexor pollicis brevis with radial sesamoid bone (cut)
8 Abductor pollicis brevis (cut)
9 Abductor digiti minimi (cut)
10 Flexor digiti minimi (cut)
11 Opponens digiti minimi
12 Flexor retinaculum (cut)
13 Pisiform bone
14 Tendon of flexor carpi ulnaris

*Shaped like a feather with a central shaft between its two vanes.

Redrawn from Wolf-Heidegger

42 Arteries of the hand

Simplified. Smaller branches are not shown

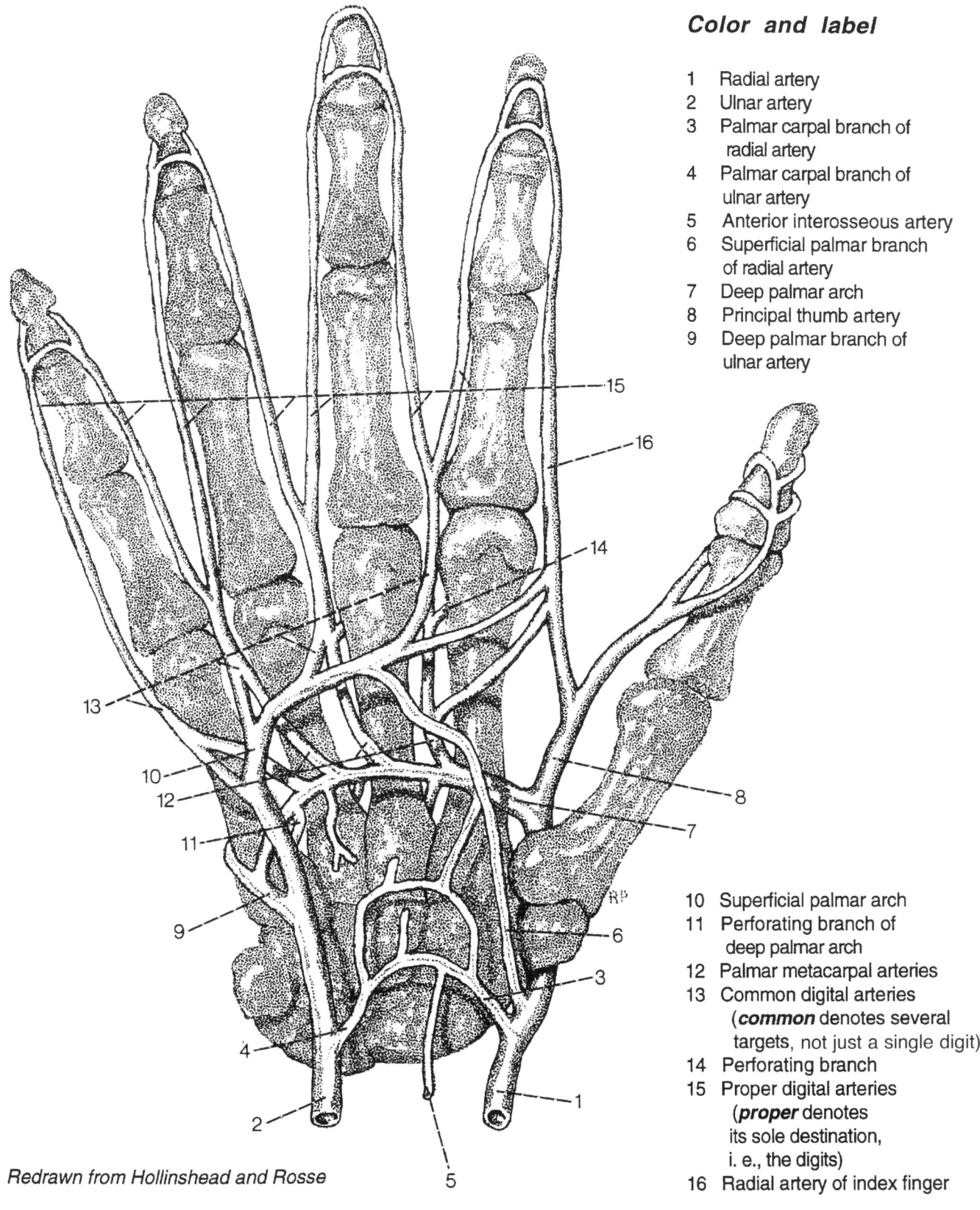

Redrawn from Hollinshead and Rosse

Color and label

1. Radial artery
2. Ulnar artery
3. Palmar carpal branch of radial artery
4. Palmar carpal branch of ulnar artery
5. Anterior interosseous artery
6. Superficial palmar branch of radial artery
7. Deep palmar arch
8. Principal thumb artery
9. Deep palmar branch of ulnar artery
10. Superficial palmar arch
11. Perforating branch of deep palmar arch
12. Palmar metacarpal arteries
13. Common digital arteries (**common** denotes several targets, not just a single digit)
14. Perforating branch
15. Proper digital arteries (**proper** denotes its sole destination, i. e., the digits)
16. Radial artery of index finger

43 Deep palmar arch and deep branch of ulnar nerve

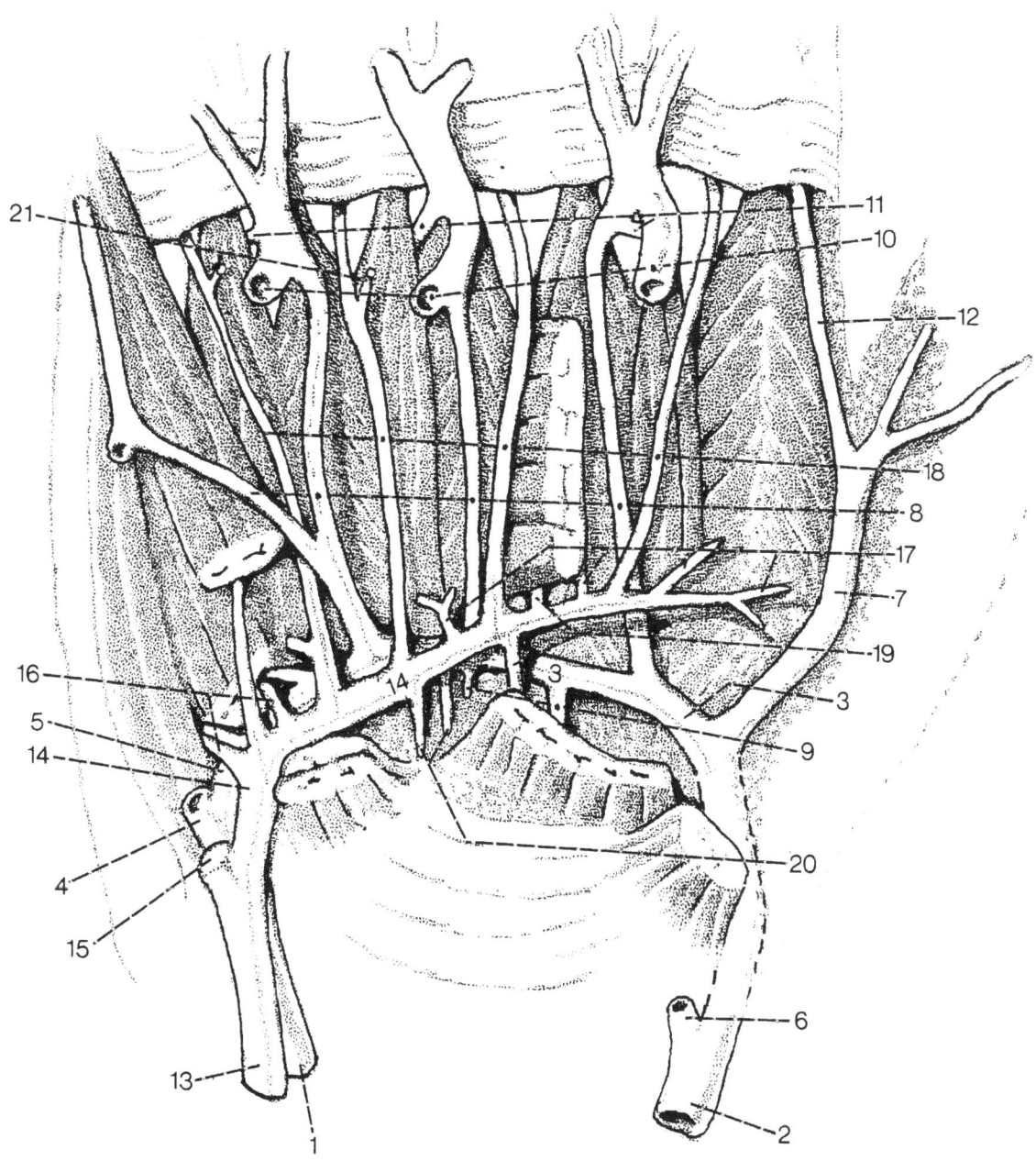

After Hollinshead and Rosse

Color and label

1. Ulnar artery
2. Radial artery
3. Deep palmar arch
4. Superficial palmar arch (cut)
5. Deep palmar branch of ulnar artery
6. Superficial palmar branch of radial artery (cut)
7. Princeps pollicis artery (main artery of the thumb)
8. Palmar metacarpal arteries
9. Perforating branches from deep palmar arch
10. Common digital arteries (cut)
11. Perforating branches of metacarpal arteries
12. Radialis indicis artery (radial artery of the index finger)
13. Ulnar nerve
14. Deep branch of ulnar nerve
15. Superficial branch of ulnar nerve (cut)
16. Ulnar nerve branches to hypothenar muscles
17. Branches to interosseous muscles
18. Articular branches to metacarpophalangeal joints
19. Branches to two heads of adductor pollicis
20. Carpal twigs to carpal bones and joints
21. Nerves to two medial lumbricals

The ulnar nerve supplies the three hypothenar muscles, all seven interosseous muscles, the two heads of the adductor pollicis, the two medial lumbricals, and the deep head of the flexor pollicis brevis.

44 Nerves and arteries of the palm

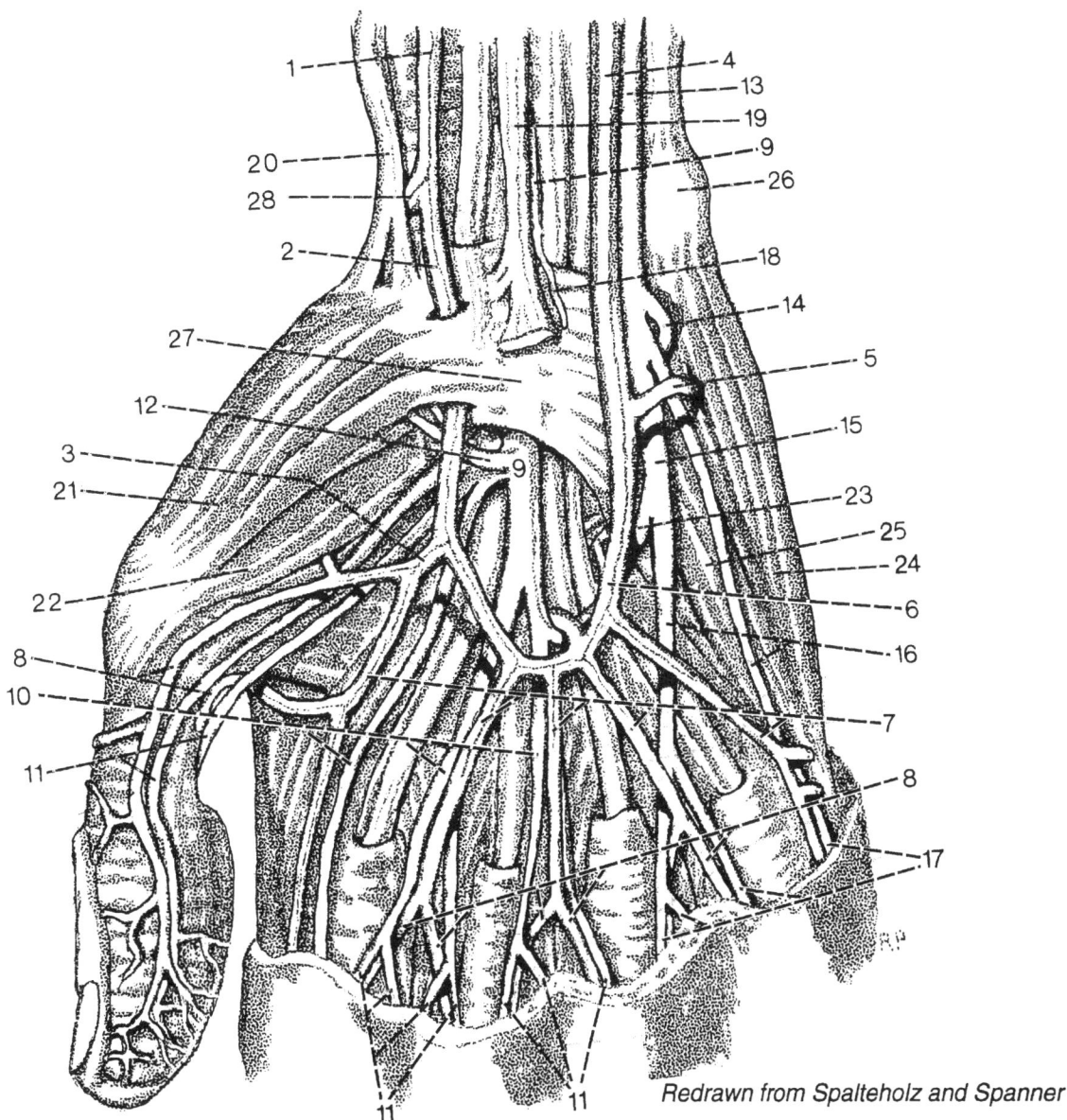

Redrawn from Spalteholz and Spanner

Color and label

1. Radial artery
2. Superficial palmar branch of radial artery
3. Principal thumb artery (princeps pollicis)
4. Ulnar artery
5. Deep branch of ulnar artery
6. Superficial palmar arch
7. Common palmar digital arteries
8. Proper palmar digital arteries
9. Median nerve
10. Common palmar digital nerves (from median nerve)
11. Proper palmar digital nerves (from median nerve)
12. Thenar muscular branch of median nerve (recurrent branch)
13. Ulnar nerve
14. Deep branch of ulnar nerve
15. Superficial branch of ulnar nerve
16. Common palmar digital nerves (from ulnar nerve)
17. Proper palmar digital nerves (from ulnar nerve)
18. Palmar branch of median nerve
19. Tendon of palmaris longus
20. Tendon of abductor pollicis longus
21. Abductor pollicis brevis
22. Flexor pollicis brevis
23. Communicating branch between median and ulnar nerves
24. Abductor digiti minimi
25. Flexor digiti minimi
26. Pisiform bone
27. Flexor retinaculum
28. Deep palmar branch of radial artery

45 Superficial palmar arch, median and ulnar nerves
(opposite page)

Color and label

1. Superficial palmar branch of radial artery
2. Tendon of extensor pollicis longus muscle
3. Tendon of abductor pollicis longus muscle
4. Tendon of palmaris longus muscle (cut)
5. Ulnar artery
6. Ulnar nerve
7. Flexor retinaculum (old name, transverse carpal ligament)
8. Abductor digiti minimi muscle
9. Median nerve emerging from carpal tunnel and dividing into common palmar digital nerves. The median nerve supplies sensation to the palmar surface of the thumb, index finger, middle finger, and lateral half of the ring finger; plus the dorsal surface of the distal phalanges of the same fingers.
10. Communicating branch of the ulnar nerve with the median nerve
11. Superficial palmar arch (formed by the radial and ulnar arteries)
12. Flexor tendons (superficial and deep) to fingers 2-5
13. Proper palmar digital nerves. The ulnar nerve supplies sensation to the fifth finger and the medial half of the ring finger.
14. Common palmar digital arteries. Notice how these arteries sometimes pass through the accompanying digital nerves.
15. Proper palmar digital arteries
16. Annular (ring-like) fibers of fibrous tendon sheaths. These strongly anchor the flexor tendons to the metacarpal and phalanges bones and thus prevent the tendons from bowing.
17. Cruciate (crossing) fibers of fibrous tendon sheaths. These occur at the joints of the fingers and allow the sheaths to fold when the fingers bend.
18. Adductor pollicis muscle
19. First lumbrical muscle. The median nerve usually supplies the two lateral lumbricals.
20. Flexor pollicis brevis muscle
21. Branch of the median nerve to the thenar muscles
22. Abductor pollicis brevis muscle

Redrawn from Tondury

45 Superficial palmar arch: median and ulnar nerves

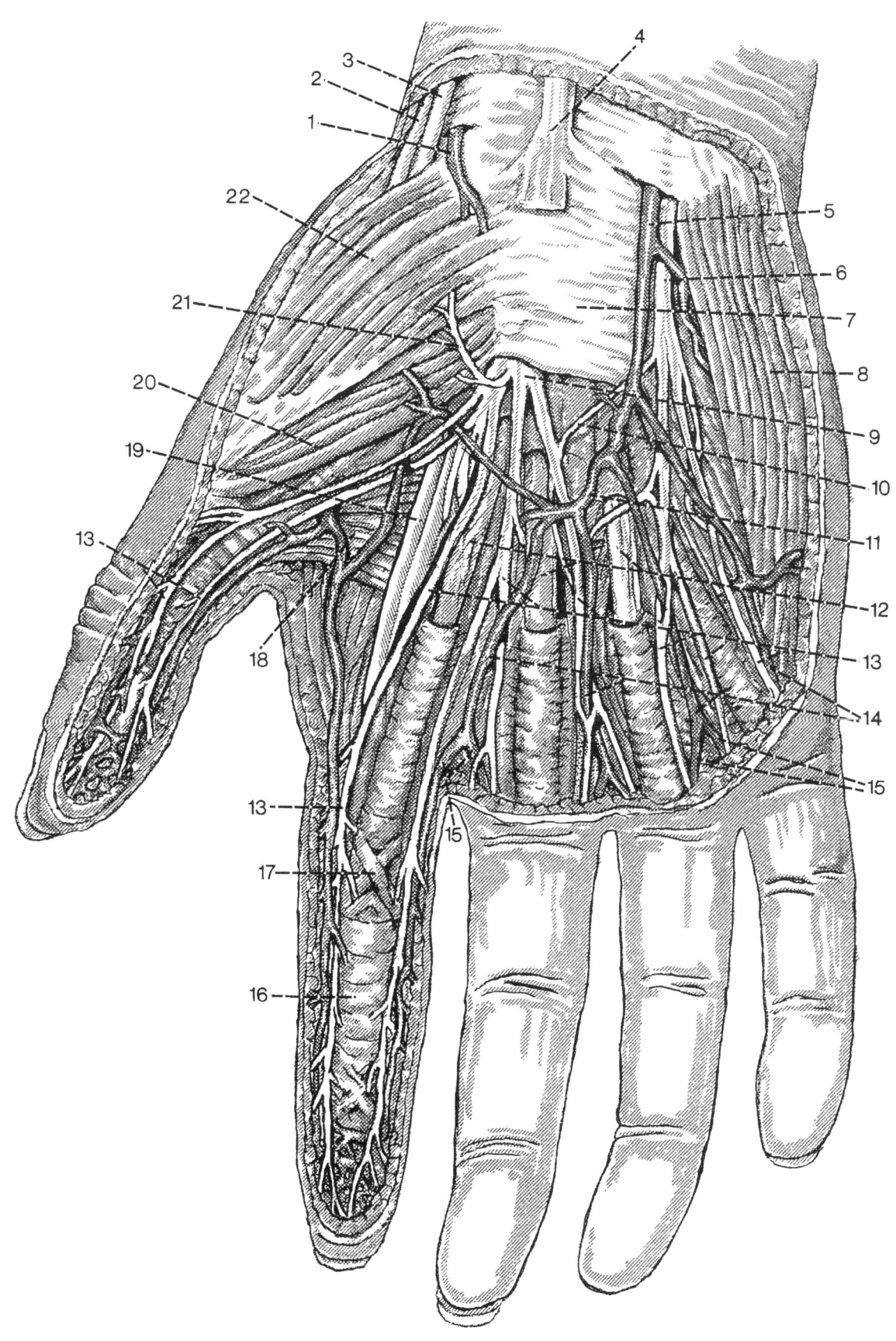

46 Extensor tendons on dorsum of hand I

(opposite page)

Color and label

1. Tendon of extensor carpi radialis longus muscle
2. Tendon of extensor carpi radialis brevis muscle; these two extensors of the wrist insert on the two strongest bones in the hand: the 2nd and 3rd metacarpals; they also stabilize the wrist by working with the finger flexors.
3. Abductor pollicis longus muscle
4. Extensor pollicis brevis muscle
5. Tendon of extensor pollicis longus muscle
6. Radius
7. Tendon of extensor pollicis brevis muscle
8. Tendon of abductor pollicis longus muscle
9. Extensor retinaculum
10. Styloid process of radius
11. Tendon of flexor carpi radialis muscle
12. First dorsal interosseous muscle
13. Adductor pollicis muscle
14. Dorsal digital expansion of the extensor digitorum tendon to the index finger
15. Four tendons of the extensor digitorum muscle
16. Extensor carpi ulnaris muscle
17. Extensor digiti minimi muscle
18. Styloid process of ulna
19. Lunate wrist bone
20. Tendon of extensor carpi ulnaris
21. Tendons of extensor digitorum muscle to fingers 2-5
22. Tendon of extensor indicis muscle to index finger
23. Tendon of extensor digiti minimi muscle; fingers 2 and 5 each have an additional extensor muscle giving them the ability to extend separately from the other fingers.
24. Dorsal interosseous muscles

Tr Trapezium wrist bone
Td Trapezoideum wrist bone
C   Capitate wrist bone
H   Hamate wrist bone
S   Scaphoid wrist bone
Tq Triquetral wrist bone

All the extensor arm muscles are innervated by the radial nerve or its posterior interosseous branch.

46 Extensor tendons on dorsum of hand I

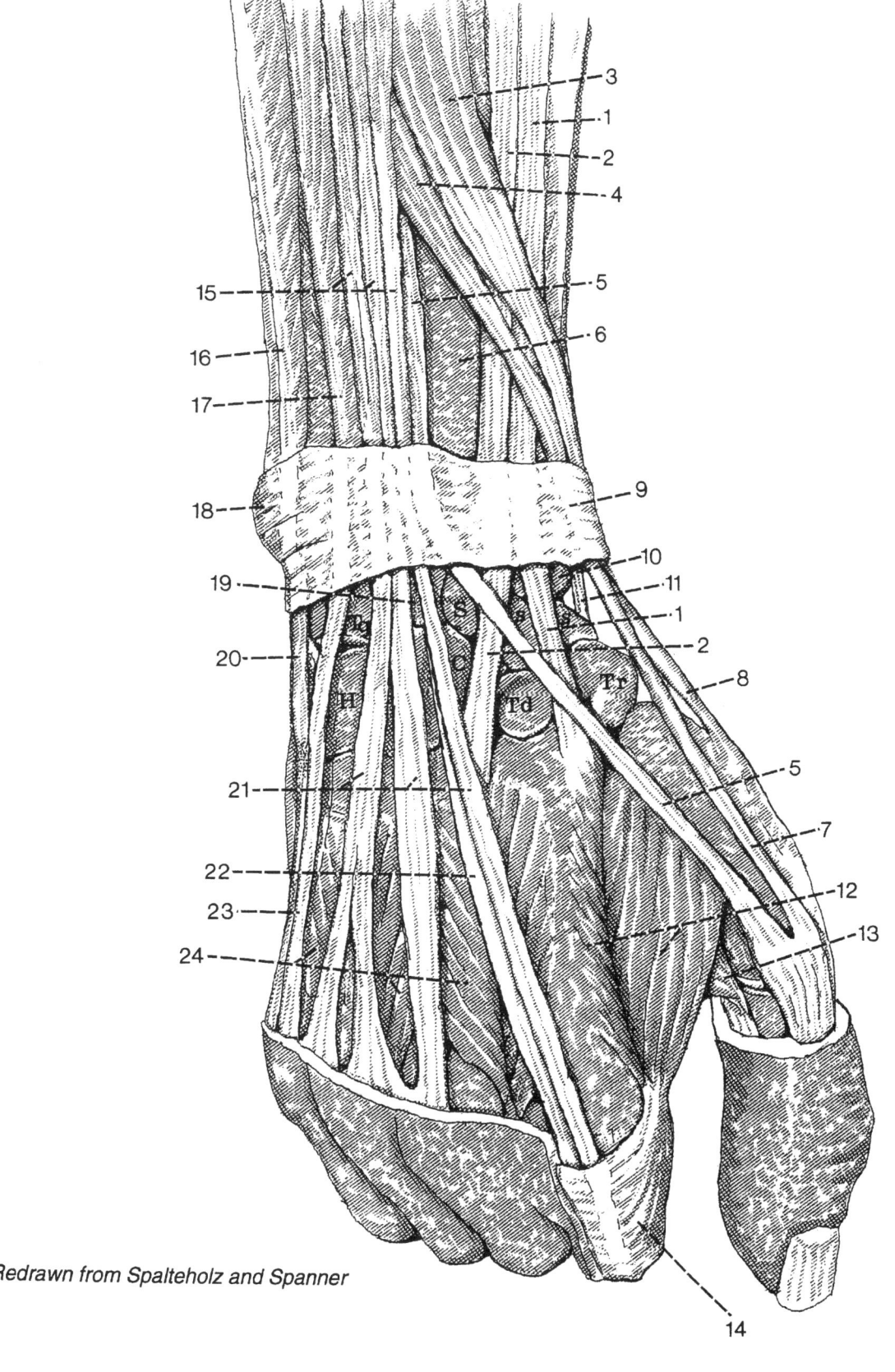

Redrawn from Spalteholz and Spanner

47 Extensor tendons on dorsum of hand II

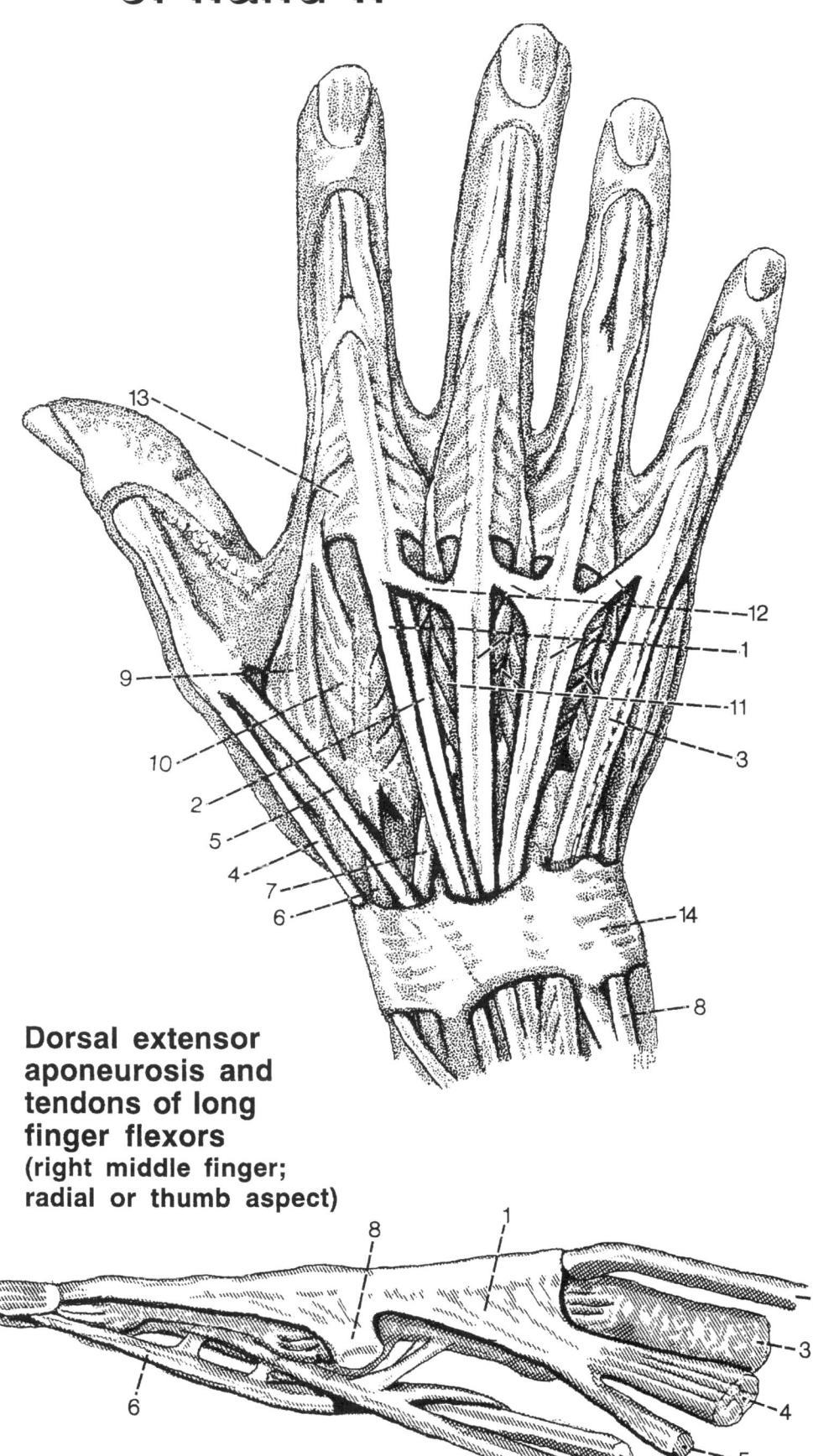

Color and label

1. Tendons of extensor digitorum to fingers 2-5
2. Tendon of extensor indicis
3. Tendon of extensor digiti minimi
4. Tendon of extensor pollicis brevis
5. Tendon of extensor pollicis longus
6. Tendon of extensor carpi radialis longus
7. Tendon of extensor carpi radialis brevis
8. Tendon of extensor of carpi ulnaris
9. First dorsal interosseous muscle (lateral head)
10. First dorsal interosseous muscle (medial head)
11. Dorsal interosseous muscles 2,3,4 *
12. Intertendinous connections
13. Dorsal extensor aponeurosis (also called dorsal digital expansion or extensor hood)
14. Extensor retinaculum

*The interossei muscles attach to both the dorsal extensor aponeurosis as well as to the proximal phalanx.

Dorsal extensor aponeurosis and tendons of long finger flexors (right middle finger; radial or thumb aspect)

Color and label

1. Dorsal extensor aponeurosis
2. Tendon of extensor digitorum
3. Metacarpal bone of middle finger
4. Dorsal interosseous muscle II
5. Lumbrical muscle II
6. Tendon of flexor digitorum profundus muscle
7. Tendon of flexor digitorum superficialis muscle
8. Cruciform (crossing) fibers of the fibrous digital sheath (cut and reflected, allowing long flexor tendons 6 and 7 to be pulled away from phalanges)

Redrawn from Wolf-Heidegger

48 Radial artery and superficial branch of radial nerve

Color and label

1. Cutaneous branch of radial nerve
2. Brachioradialis muscle
3. Tendon of flexor carpi radialis
4. Tendon of palmaris longus muscle
5. Radial artery
6. Palmar branch of median nerve
7. Median nerve
8. Tendon of abductor pollicis longus muscle
9. Superficial palmar branch of radial artery
10. Opponens pollicis muscle
11. Abductor pollicis muscle
12. Extensor pollicis brevis tendon
13. Extensor pollicis longus tendon. Notice that these two extensor tendons of the thumb define the anatomical "snuff box", through which traverses the radial artery.
14. First dorsal interosseous muscle.
15. First metacarpal bone
16. Thumb (digit 1)
17. Index finger (digit 2)
18. Second metacarpal bone
19. Cutaneous branch of radial nerve
20. Superficial branch of radial nerve
21. Extensor pollicis brevis muscle
22. Extensor retinaculum
23. Extensor carpi radialis brevis tendon (inserts on 3rd metacarpal)
24. Extensor carpi radialis longus tendon (inserts on 2nd metacarpal)
25. First dorsal metacarpal artery

Redrawn from Tondury

49 Dorsum of hand
(opposite page)

After removal of fascia and dorsal venous plexus

Color and label

1. Superficial branch of radial nerve
2. Cutaneous branch of radial nerve
3. Extensor retinaculum
4. Extensor carpi radialis longus tendon
5. Radial artery
6. Extensor carpi radialis brevis tendon
7. Dorsal metacarpal artery
8. Connection between dorsal cutaneous branches of radial and ulnar nerves
9. Extensor pollicis longus tendon
10. First dorsal interosseous muscle
11. Extensor indicis tendon
12. Dorsal digital nerves
13. Dorsal digital expansion; a triangular aponeurotic extension of each of the four tendons of the extensor digitorum on the proximal phalanges of digits 2-5. They each serve as an attachment for the lumbricals and the interosseous muscles.
14. Dorsal digital veins (cut; veins have been largely removed)
15. Extensor digiti minimi tendon
16. Four tendons of extensor digitorum to digits 2-5
17. Dorsal ramus of ulnar nerve
18. Dorsal antebrachial rami of radial nerve
19. Venous network on dorsum of hand; (cut); these coalesce and drain proximally mainly into the cephalic vein (thumb side) and basilic vein (little finger side).

Redrawn from Tondury

49 Dorsum of hand

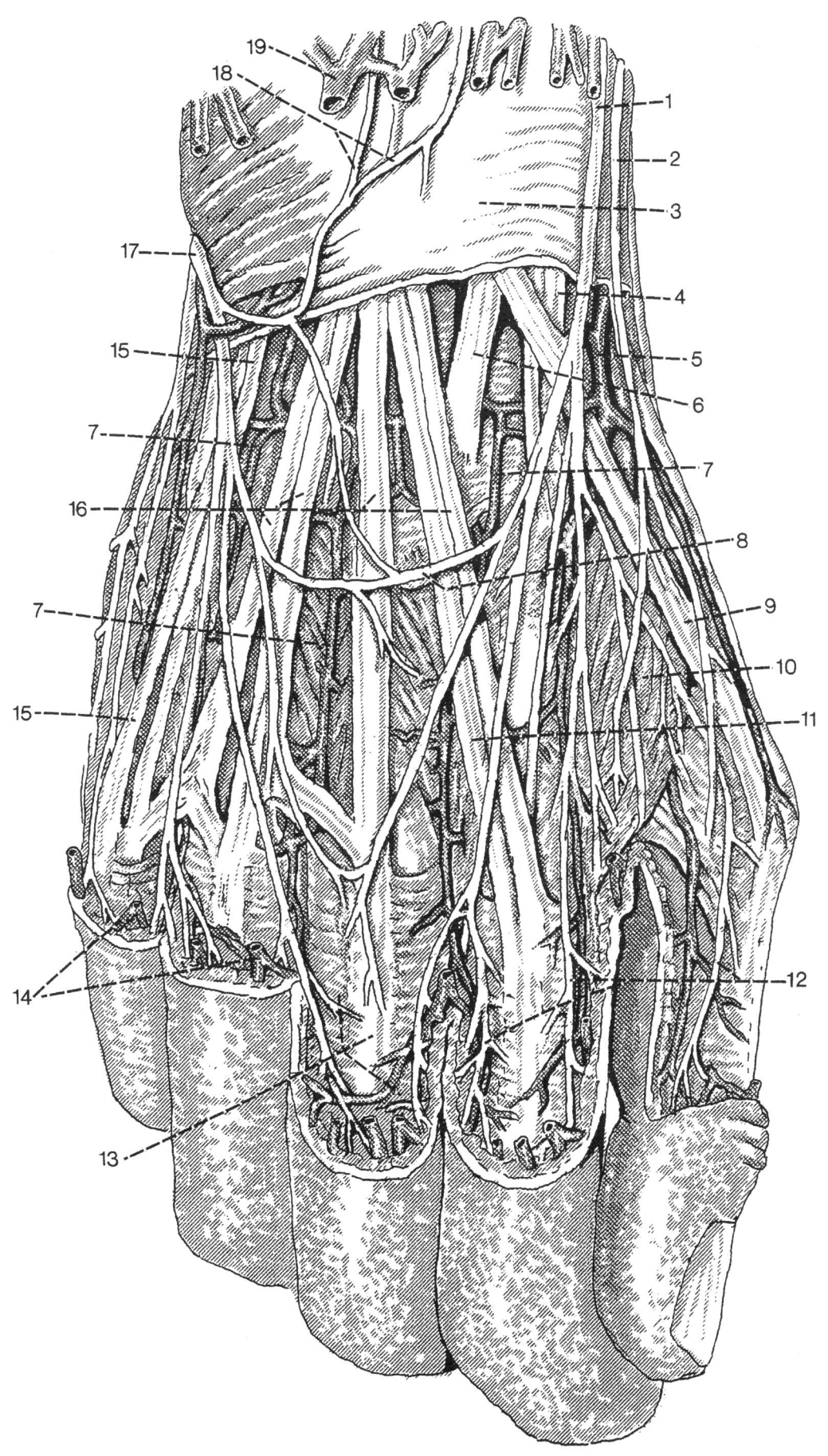

50 Palmar hand: deep dissection
(opposite page)

Color and label

1. Tendon of palmaris longus
2. Ulnar artery
3. Ulnar nerve
4. Flexor retinaculum
5. Deep palmar branch of ulnar artery
6. Four tendons of flexor digitorum superficialis muscle
7. Four tendons of flexor digitorum profundus muscle
8. Deep branch of ulnar nerve to interosseous muscle
9. Opponens digiti minimi muscle
10. Abductor digiti minimi muscle
11. Flexor digiti minimi brevis muscle
12. Palmar metacarpal arteries
13. Tendon of flexor digitorum profundus of 5th finger (cut)
14. Tendon of flexor digitorum superficialis of 5th finger (cut)
15. Proper digital artery of 5th finger (cut)
16. Proper digital nerve of 5th finger (cut)
17. Adductor pollicis muscle transverse head (cut)
18. Adductor pollicis muscle oblique head (cut)
19. Adductor pollicis muscle insertion (cut)
20. Tendon of flexor pollicis longus muscle (in sheath)
21. Flexor pollicis brevis muscle superficial head (cut)
22. Flexor pollicis brevis muscle deep head
23. Abductor pollicis brevis muscle (cut)
24. Principal thumb artery (off radial artery)
25. Opponens pollicis muscle (partially cut in half)
26. Radial artery origin of deep palmar arch
27. Median nerve (divisions cut)
28. Abductor pollicis muscle origin on flexor retinaculum
29. Lumbrical muscles (to third and fourth fingers)

P   Palmar interosseous muscles
D   Dorsal interosseous muscles

50 Palmar hand: deep dissection

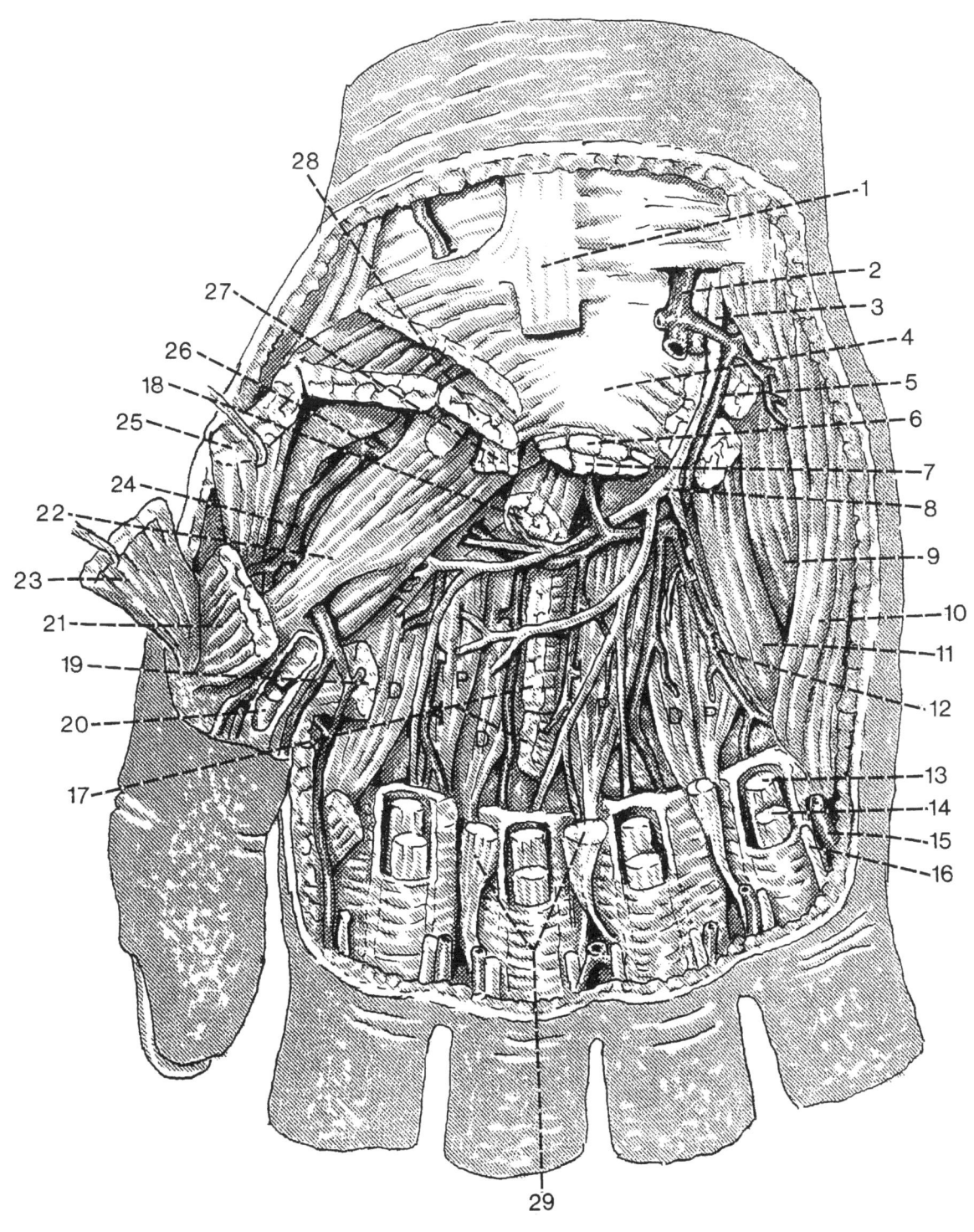

Redrawn from Tondury

51 Synovial flexor tendon sheaths

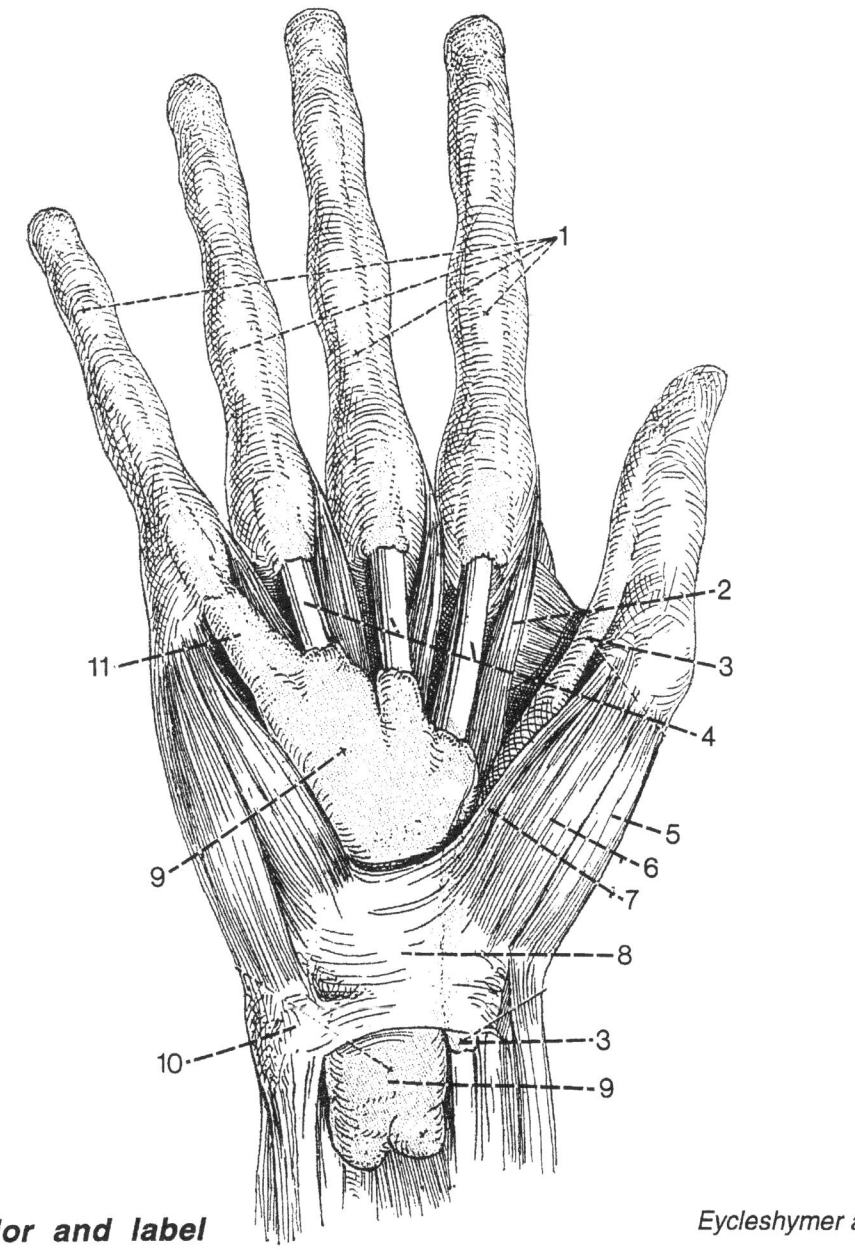

Color and label

Eycleshymer and Jones

1. Digital synovial tendon sheaths; these are surrounded by the fibrous tendon sheaths.
2. First lumbrical muscle
3. Synovial tendon sheath for flexor pollicis longus; note its separation from the common synovial sheath
4. Flexor tendons (deep and superficial) to fingers 2,3,4
5. Opponens pollicis muscle
6. Abductor pollicis brevis muscle
7. Flexor pollicis brevis muscle
8. Flexor retinaculum
9. Common synovial sheath for flexors to fingers 2,3,4,5
10. Pisiform bone
11. Abductor digiti minimi synovial sheath; note its continuity with the common synovial sheath.

52 Synovial extensor tendon sheaths

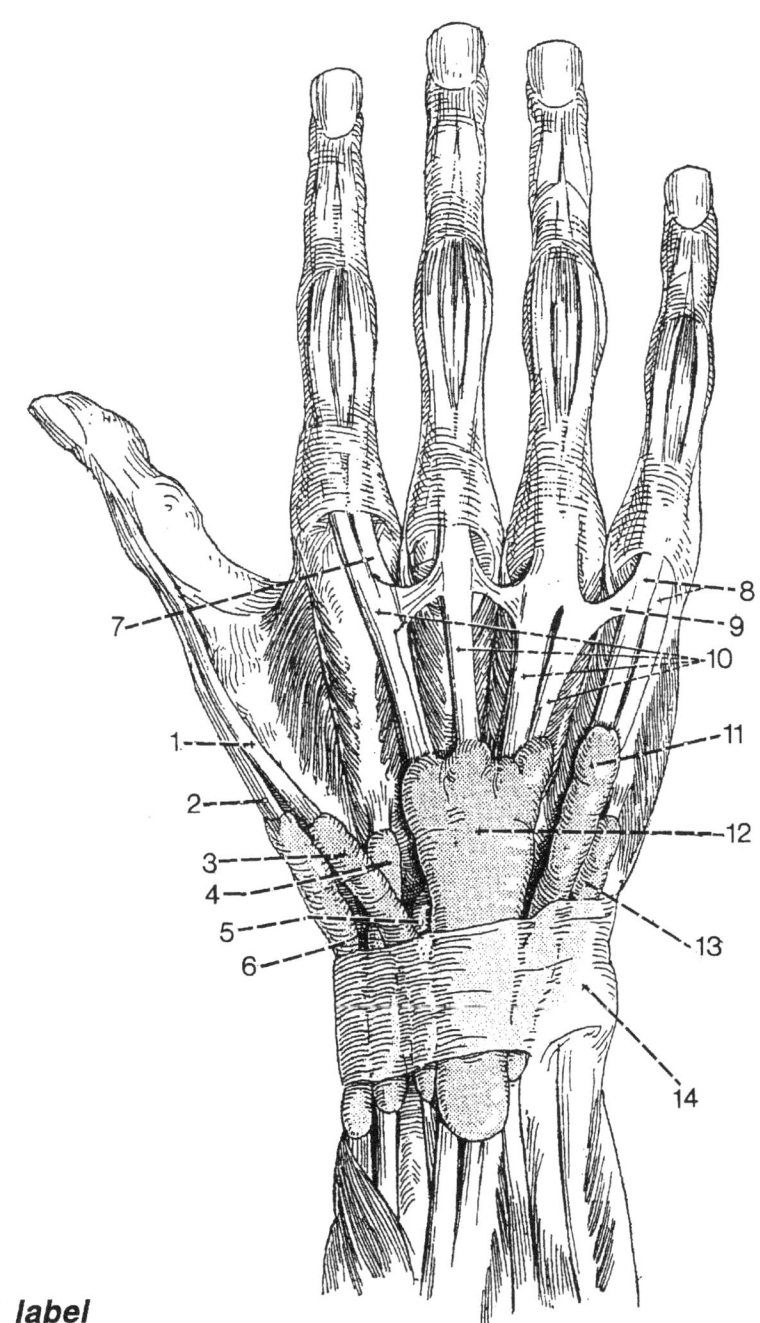

Color and label

1. Tendon of extensor pollicis longus
2. Tendon of extensor pollicis brevis
3. Extensor pollicis longus synovial tendon sheath
4. Extensor carpi radialis longus synovial tendon sheath
5. Extensor carpi radialis brevis synovial tendon sheath
6. Extensor pollicis brevis synovial tendon sheath
7. Tendon of extensor indicis
8. Tendon of extensor digiti minimi
   Notice these two "extra" extensor tendons to fingers 2 and 5 lie on the ulnar (or medial) sides of the two corresponding extensor digitorum tendons and impart an additional extensor independence to these two digits.
9. Intertendinous connection
10. Extensor digitorum tendons to fingers 2-5. Its action on finger 5 is usually conveyed via an intertendinous link to extensor digiti minimi tendon.
11. Synovial tendon sheath of extensor digiti minimi
12. Synovial tendon sheath for extensor digitorum and extensor indicis
13. Synovial tendon sheath for extensor carpi ulnaris
14. Extensor retinaculum

Eycleshymer and Jones

53 Thumb muscles I

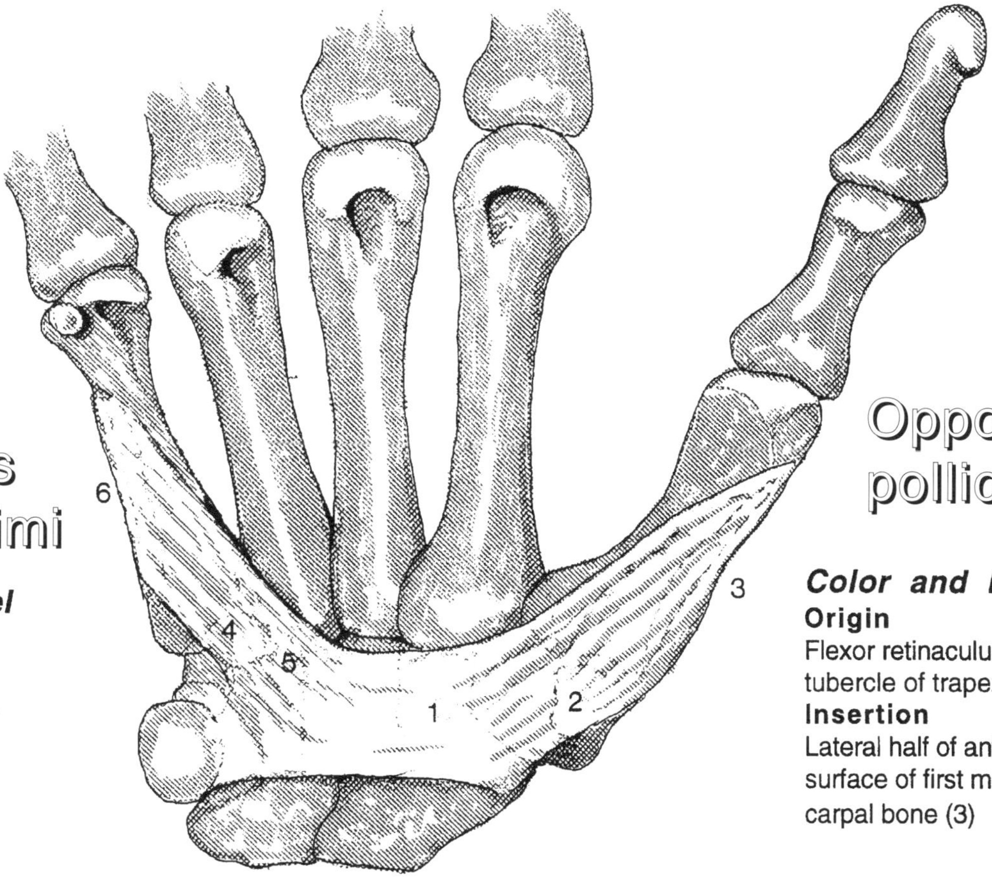

Opponens digiti minimi

Color and label

Origin
Distal margin of hook of the hamate (4) and its adjacent flexor retinaculum (5)

Insertion
Medial margin of 5th metacarpal bone (6)

Opponens pollicis

Color and label

Origin
Flexor retinaculum (1) and tubercle of trapezium (2)

Insertion
Lateral half of anterior surface of first metacarpal bone (3)

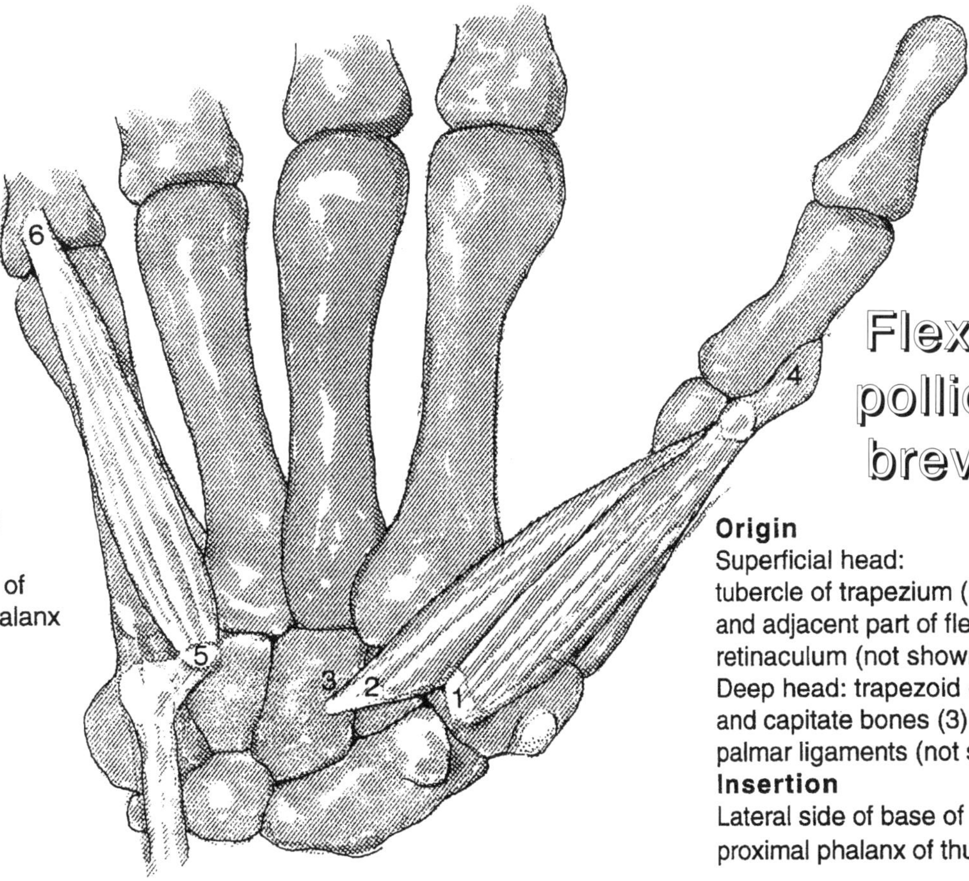

Flexor digiti minimi

Origin
Hook of hamate (5)

Insertion
Medial side of base of base of proximal phalanx of little finger (6)

Flexor pollicis brevis

Origin
Superficial head: tubercle of trapezium (1) and adjacent part of flexor retinaculum (not shown)
Deep head: trapezoid (2) and capitate bones (3) and palmar ligaments (not shown)

Insertion
Lateral side of base of proximal phalanx of thumb (4)

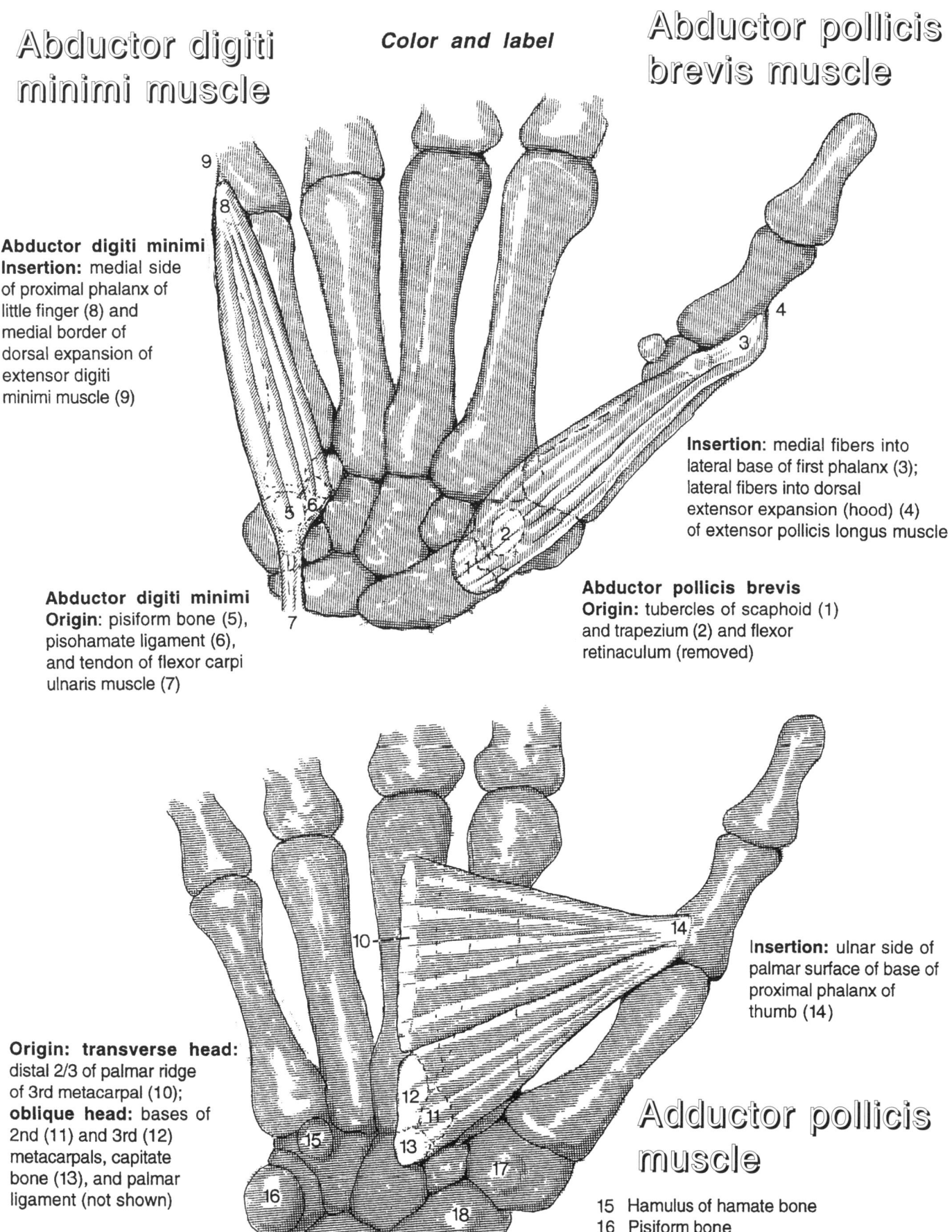

55 Palmar interosseous muscles

Palmar aspect of right hand

Redrawn from Spalteholz and Spanner

ADDUCTION

Color and label

1. First palmar interosseous muscle
2. Second palmar interosseous muscle
3. Third palmar interosseous muscle
4. Radius
5. Ulna
6. Lumbrical muscles (cut)
7. Fibrous tendon sheaths for superficial and deep flexor tendons (cut open and tendons removed)
8. Pisiform bone
9. Hook of hamate bone
10. First dorsal interosseous muscle (cut)

The palmar interosseous muscles, usually described as consisting of three muscles, as depicted here, are described by some authors as consisting of four muscles. According to these authors*, the first palmar interosseous, which is usually considered part of either the flexor pollicis or the adductor pollicis arises from the medial side of the palmar surface of first metacarpal bone near its base (not shown here). The present account depicts three palmar interosseous muscles rather than four. The first arises from the medial surface of the second metacarpal and inserts into the medial side of the base of the proximal phalange and the medial side of the dorsal digital expansion of the index finger. The second arises from the lateral surface of the fourth metacarpal and inserts onto the lateral side of the dorsal digital expansion of the ring finger. The third arises from the lateral side of the fifth metacarpal and inserts into the lateral side of the dosal digital expansion of the fifth finger. The palmar interossei **adduct** the 2nd, 4th, and fifth fingers toward the middle finger. They also flex the proximal phalanx and extend the middle phalanx and distal phalanx of the four medial fingers.

*Gray's Anatomy, 38th ed., 1995, Edinburgh, Churchill Livingstone

56 Dorsal interosseous muscles of the hand

Dorsal aspect right hand

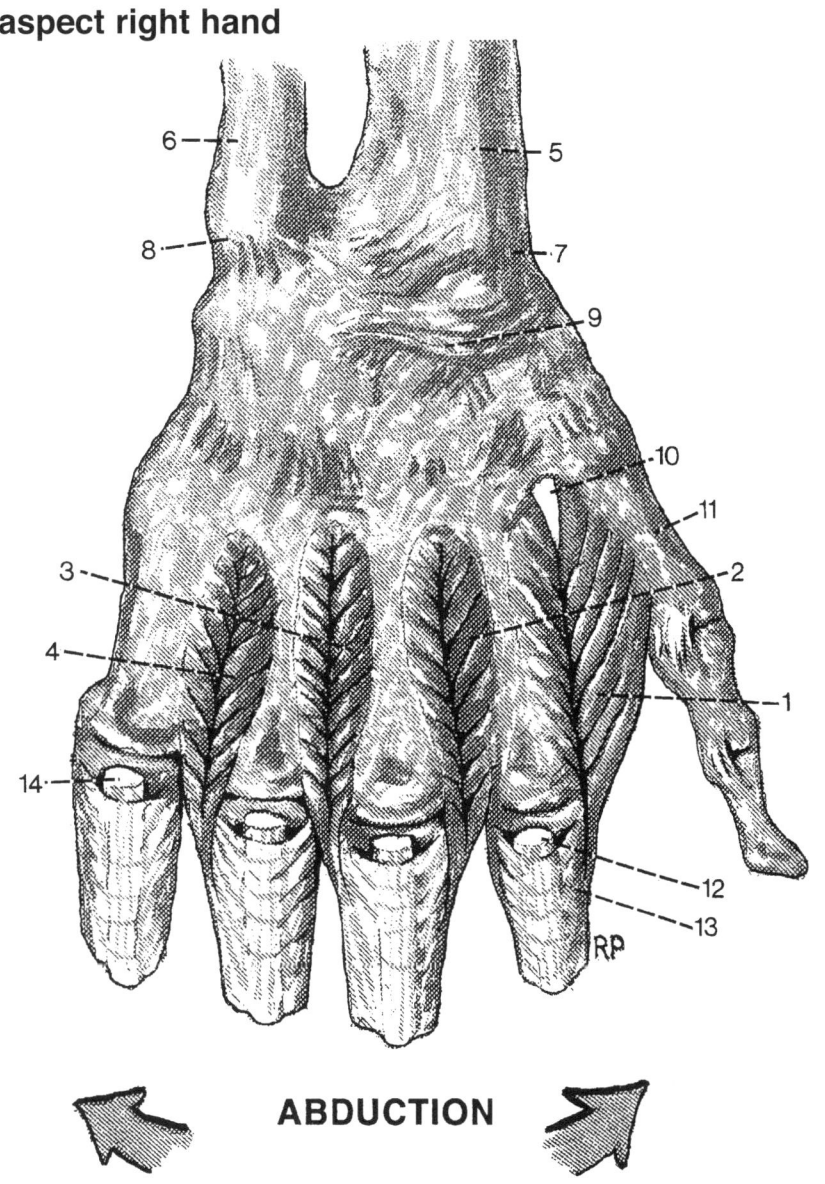

ABDUCTION

Color and label

1. First dorsal interosseous
2. Second dorsal interosseous
3. Third dorsal interosseous
4. Fourth dorsal interosseous
5. Radius
6. Ulna
7. Styloid process of radius
8. Styloid process of ulna
9. Dorsal intercarpal ligaments
10. Foramen for radial artery
11. First carpal bone (of thumb)
12. Extensor digitorum tendon of index finger (cut)
13. Dorsal digital expansion of extensor tendon of index finger
14. Extensor digitorum tendon of little finger (digiti minimi) (cut)

The dorsal interosseous muscles are four bipennate muscles in each hand. They each arise from adjacent sides of two metacarpal bones and insert onto the bases of proximal phalanges and dorsal digital (extensor tendon) expansions. The first inserts on the radial side of the index finger. The second and third on the radial and ulnar sides, respectively, of the middle finger. The fourth inserts onto the ulnar side of the ring finger (4th). They are innervated by the deep branch of the ulnar nerve. They **abduct** the second and fourth fingers from the midline axis in the middle finger. They flex the proximal phalanges (MP joint) and extend the middle (PIP joint) and distal phalanges (DIP joint).

57 Some finger movements

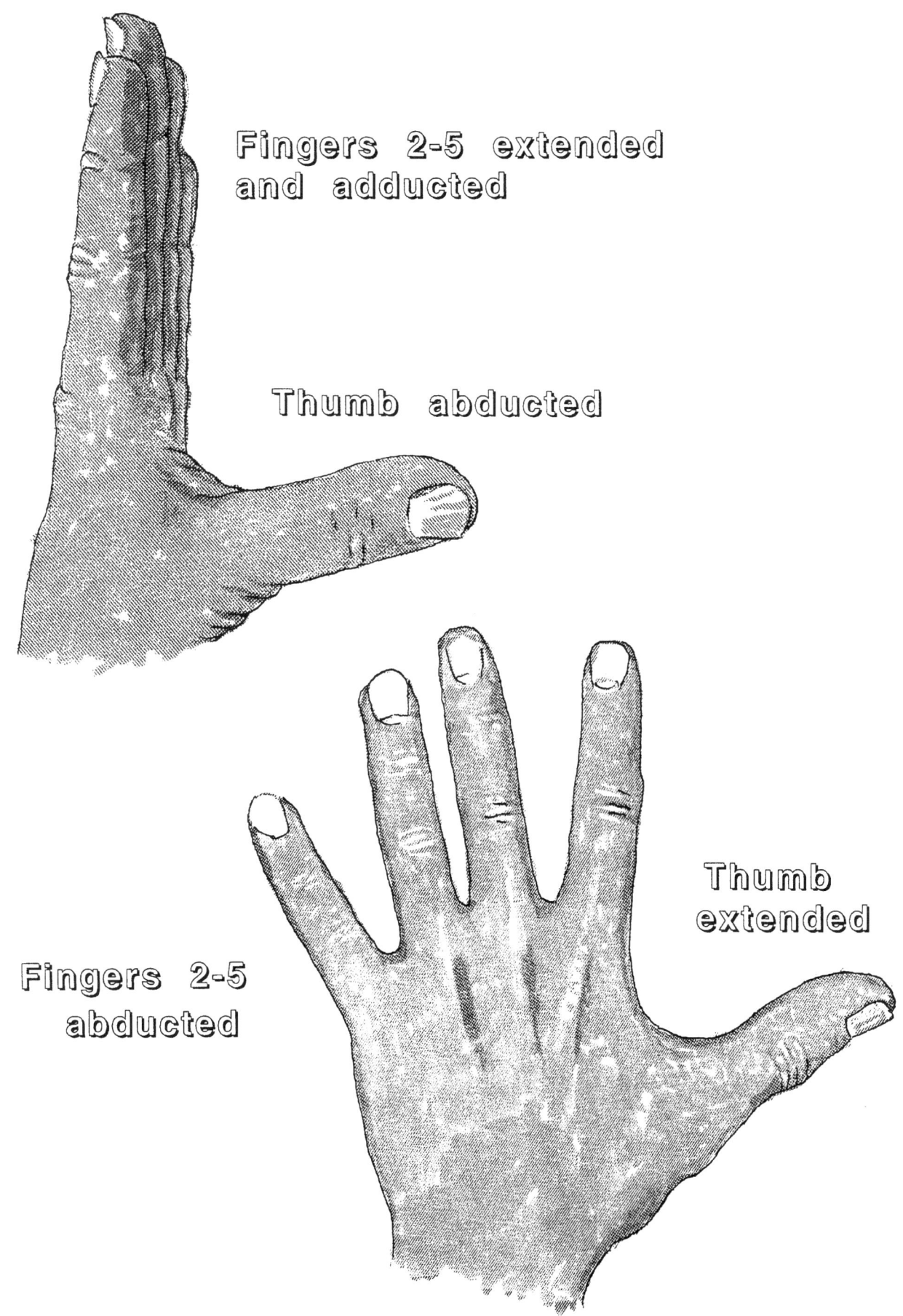

58 Cutaneous nerve distribution on front of arm

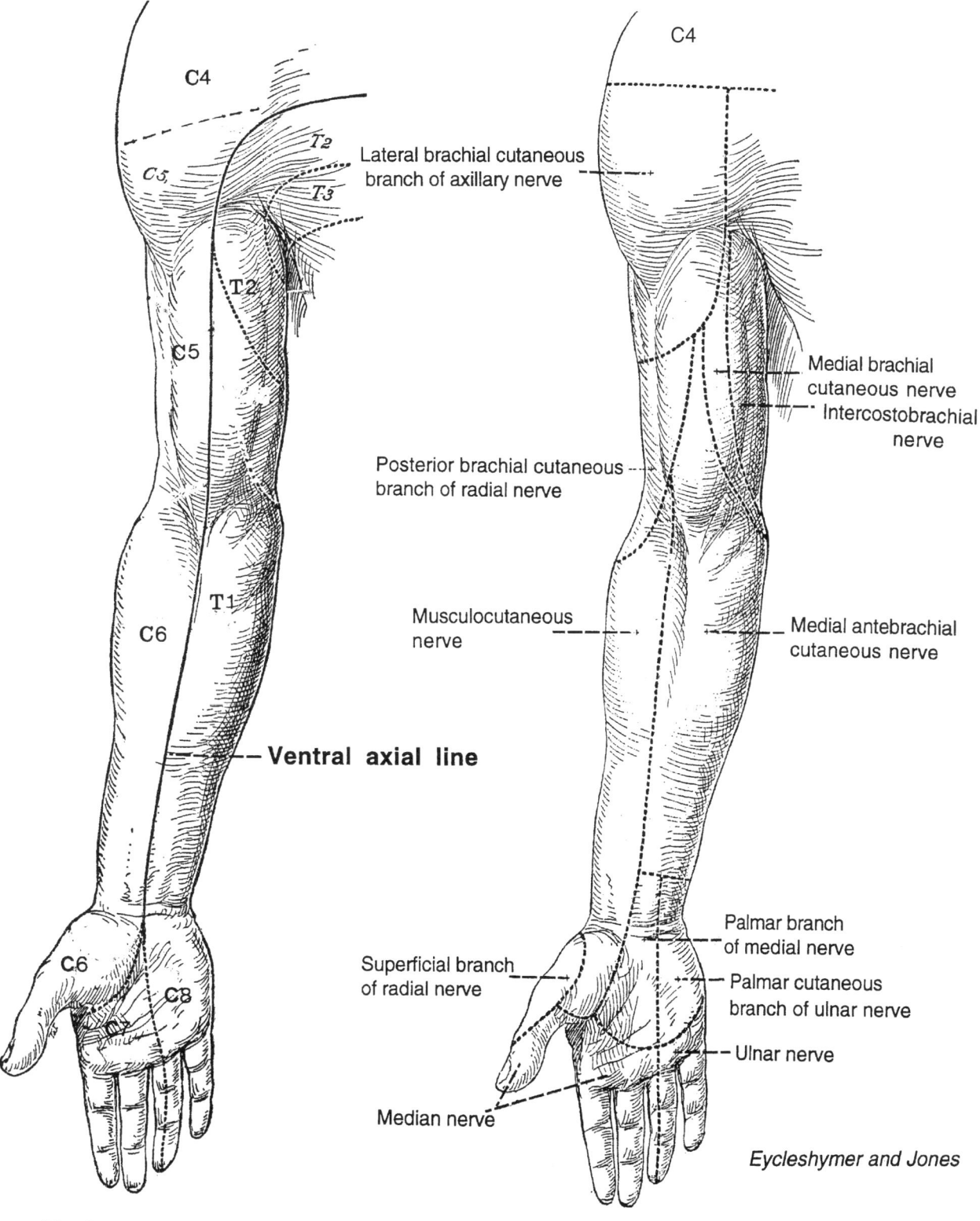

The figure on the left shows the segmental cutaneous distribution of the **principal** cervical (C) and thoracic (T) spinal nerves to the skin of the anterior arm. There is considerable overlap from adjacent spinal nerves both above and below the indicated nerve level. However, there is very little overlap of the vertral axial line. The figure on the right shows the areas of distribution of the cutaneous nerves.

59 Distribution of cutaneous nerves on back of upper limb

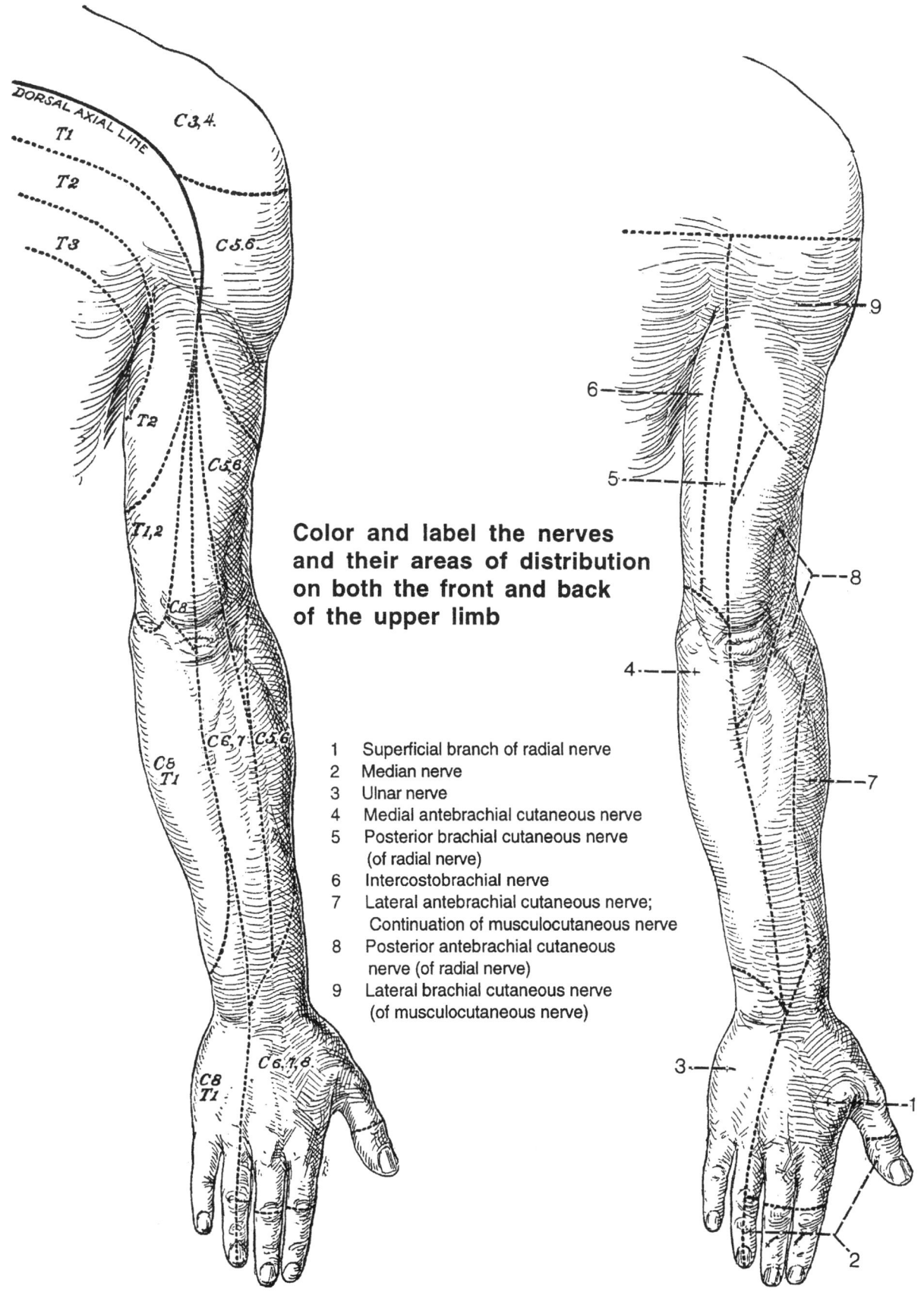

Color and label the nerves and their areas of distribution on both the front and back of the upper limb

1. Superficial branch of radial nerve
2. Median nerve
3. Ulnar nerve
4. Medial antebrachial cutaneous nerve
5. Posterior brachial cutaneous nerve (of radial nerve)
6. Intercostobrachial nerve
7. Lateral antebrachial cutaneous nerve; Continuation of musculocutaneous nerve
8. Posterior antebrachial cutaneous nerve (of radial nerve)
9. Lateral brachial cutaneous nerve (of musculocutaneous nerve)

60 Muscle attachments of the anterior arm

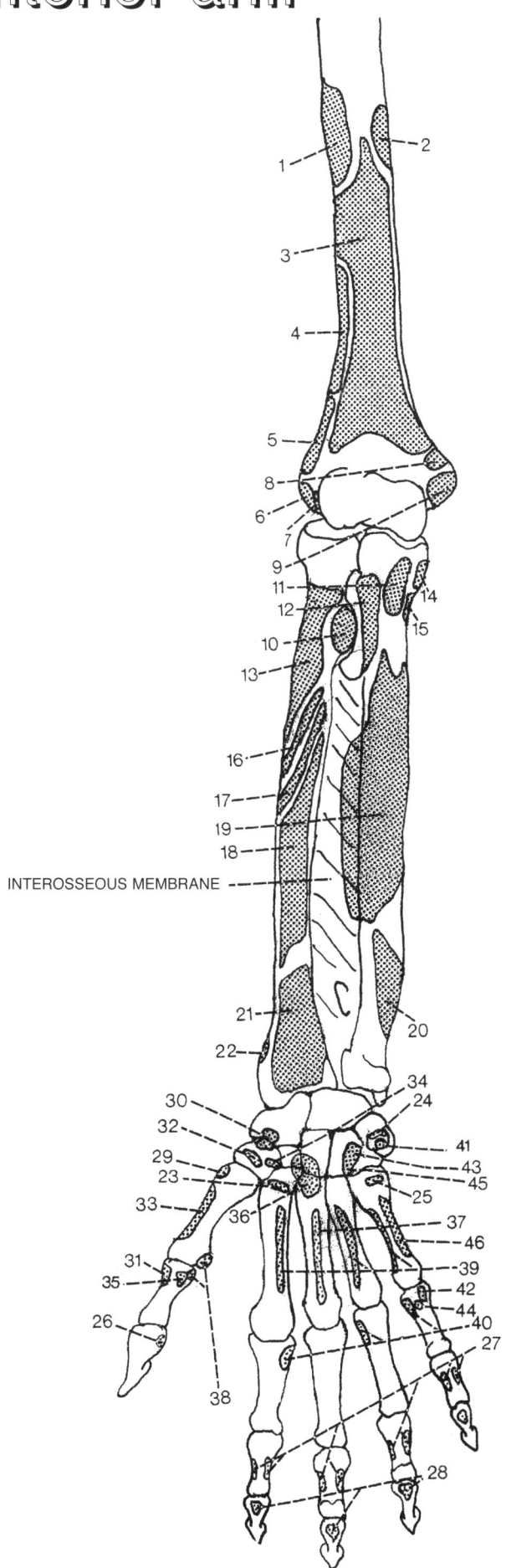

Color the origins (O) RED and the insertions (I) BLUE

1. Deltoid (I)
2. Coracobrachialis (I)
3. Brachialis (O)
4. Brachioradialis (O)
5. Extensor carpi radialis longus (O)
6. Extensor carpi radialis brevis (O) and extensor digitorum (O)
7. Supinator (O), humeral part
8. Pronator teres (O), humeral head
9. Common origin for flexor carpi radialis, palmaris longus, flexor carpi ulnaris, flexor digitorum superficialis (O)
10. Biceps brachii (I)
11. Brachialis (I)
12. Supinator (O), ulnar part
13. Supinator (I)
14. Flexor digitorum superficialis (O), ulnar origin
15. Pronator teres (O), ulnar head
16. Pronator teres (I)
17. Flexor digitorum superficialis (O), radial origin
18. Flexor pollicis longus (O)
19. Flexor digitorum profundus (O)
20. Pronator quadratus (O)
21. Pronator quadratus (I)
22. Brachioradialis (I)
23. Flexor carpi radialis (I)
24. Flexor carpi ulnaris insertion on pisiform bone (I)
25. Flexor carpi ulnaris insertion on 5th metacarpal (I)
26. Flexor pollicis longus (I)
27. Flexor digitorum superficialis (I)
28. Flexor digitorum profundus (I)
29. Abductor pollicis longus (I)
30. Abductor pollicis brevis (O)
31. Abductor pollicis brevis (I)
32. Opponens pollicis (O)
33. Opponens pollicis (I)
34. Flexor pollicis brevis (O)
35. Flexor pollicis brevis (I)
36. Adductor pollicis (O), oblique head
37. Adductor pollicis (O), transverse head
38. Adductor pollicis (I)
39. Palmar interosseous (O)
40. Palmar interosseous (I)
41. Abductor digiti minimi (O)
42. Abductor digiti minimi (I)
43. Flexor digiti minimi brevis (O)
44. Flexor digiti minimi brevis (I)
45. Opponens digiti minimi (O)
46. Opponens digiti minimi (I)

61 Muscle attachments of the posterior arm

Color the origins (O) RED and the insertions (I) BLUE

1. Sternocleidomastoid (O)
2. Pectoralis major (O)
3. Deltoid (O)
4. Trapezius (I)
5. Omohyoid (O)
6. Supraspinatus (O)
7. Levator scapulae (I)
8. Rhombold minor (I)
9. Rhomboid major (I)
10. Infraspinatus (O)
11. Teres major (O)
12. Teres minor (O)
13. Deltoid (I)
14. Infraspinatus (I)
15. Teres minor (I)
16. Triceps brachii lateral head (O)
17. Triceps brachii long head (O)
18. Triceps brachii medial head (O)
19. Anconeus (O)
20. Flexor carpi ulnaris (O)
21. Triceps brachii (I)
22. Anconeus (I)
23. Flexor digitorum superficialis (O)
24. Flexor digitorum profundus (O)
25. Supinator (O)
26. Abductor pollicis longus (O)
27. Extensor pollicis longus (O)
28. Extensor indicis (O)
29. Supinator (I)
30. Pronator teres (I)
31. Extensor pollicis brevis (I)
32. Common aponeurosis for origin of extensor carpi ulnaris, flexor carpi ulnaris, flexor digitorum profundus
33. Extensor carpi ulnaris (I)
34. Extensor carpi radialis longus (I)
35. Extensor carpi radialis brevis (I)
36. First dorsal interosseous (O)
37. Second dorsal interosseous (O)
38. Third dorsal interosseous (O)
39. Fourth dorsal interosseous (O)
40. Extensor pollicis brevis (I)
41. Extensor pollicis longus (I)
42. First dorsal interosseous (I)
43. Second dorsal interosseous (I)
44. Third dorsal interosseous (I)
45. Fourth dorsal interosseous (I)
46. Extensor digitorum (I)
47. Extensor indicis (I) (common insertion)
48. Extensor digiti minimi (common insertion)

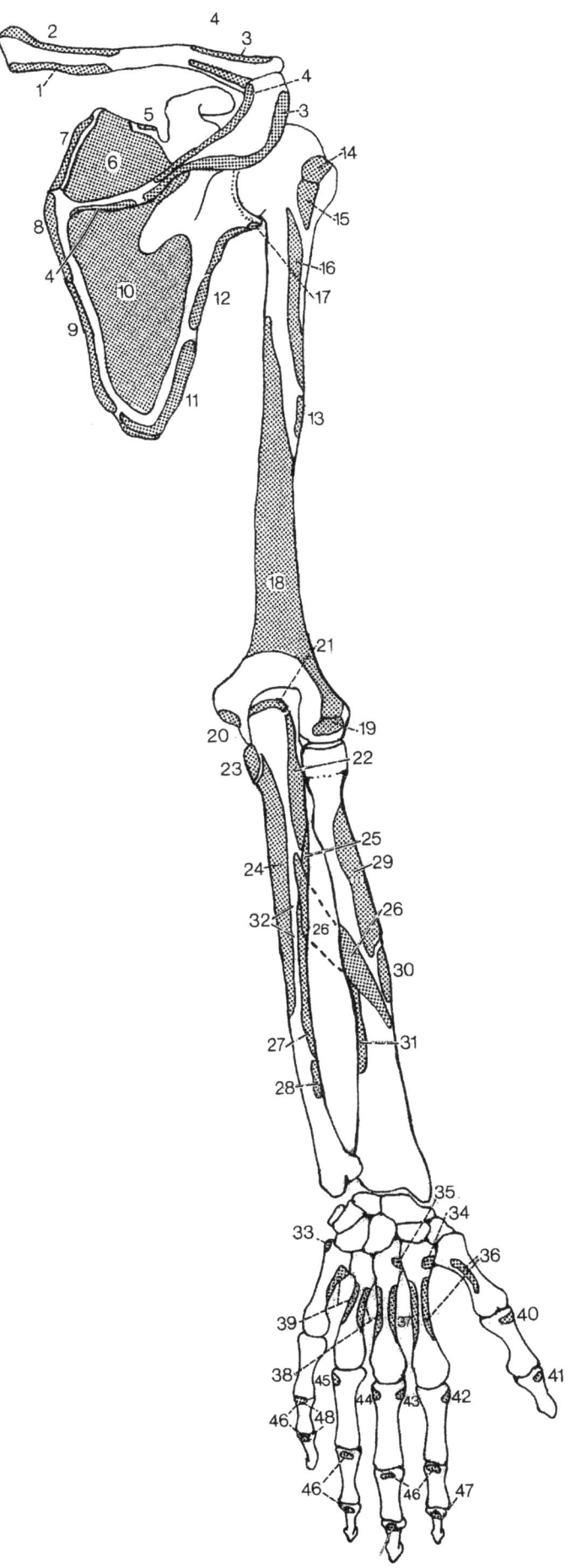

62 Muscle attachments of the anterior hand

Color the origins (O) RED and the insertions (I) BLUE

1. Adductor pollicis brevis (O)
2. Opponens pollicis (O)
3. Opponens pollicis (I)
4. Flexor pollicis brevis (O)
5. Flexor pollicis brevis and adductor pollicis brevis common sesamoid bone and insertion (I)
6. Adductor pollicis *(oblique head)* (O)
7. Adductor pollicis *(transverse head)* (O)
8. Adductor pollicis sesamoid bone and insertion (I)
9. Dorsal interosseous (1, 2, 3, 4) (O)
10. Dorsal interosseous (1, 2, 3, 4) inserts on on "hood" of extensor tendons (I)
11. Palmar (ventral) interosseous (1, 2, 3) (O)
12. Palmar (ventral) interosseous (1, 2, 3) (I)
13. Flexor digiti minimi (O) and pisohamate ligament
14. Abductor digiti minimi (O)
15. Opponens digiti minimi (O)
16. Opponens digiti minimi (I)
17. Abductor digiti minimi (I)
18. Flexor digiti minimi (I)
19. Abductor pollicis longus (I)
20. Flexor carpi radialis (I)
21. Flexor carpi ulnaris (I)
22. Flexor pollicis longus (I)
23. Flexor digitorum superficialis (I)
24. Flexor digitorum profundus (I)
25. Extensor carpi ulnaris (I) and pisometacarpal ligament

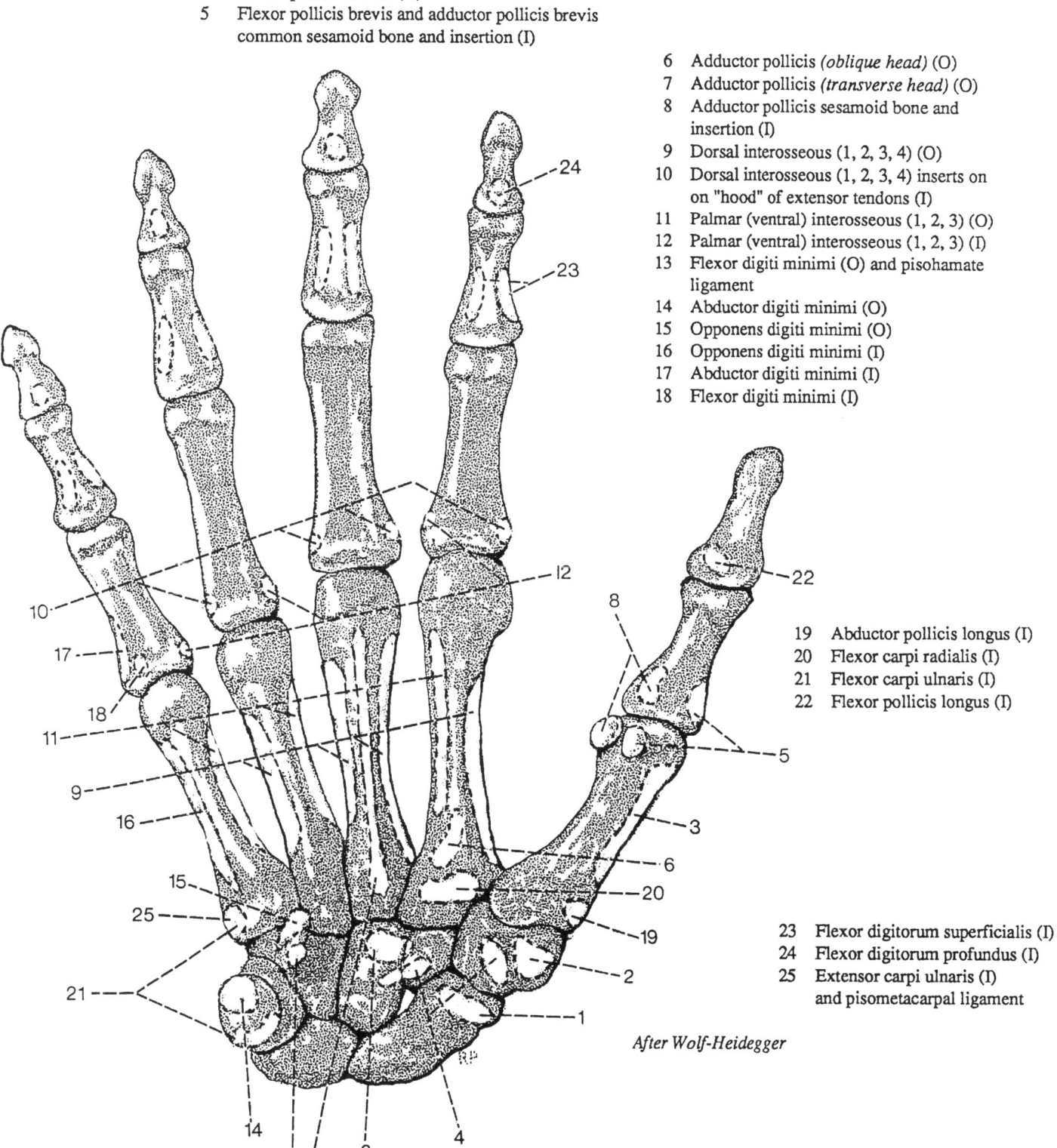

After Wolf-Heidegger

63 Frontal (coronal) section of the right wrist and hand

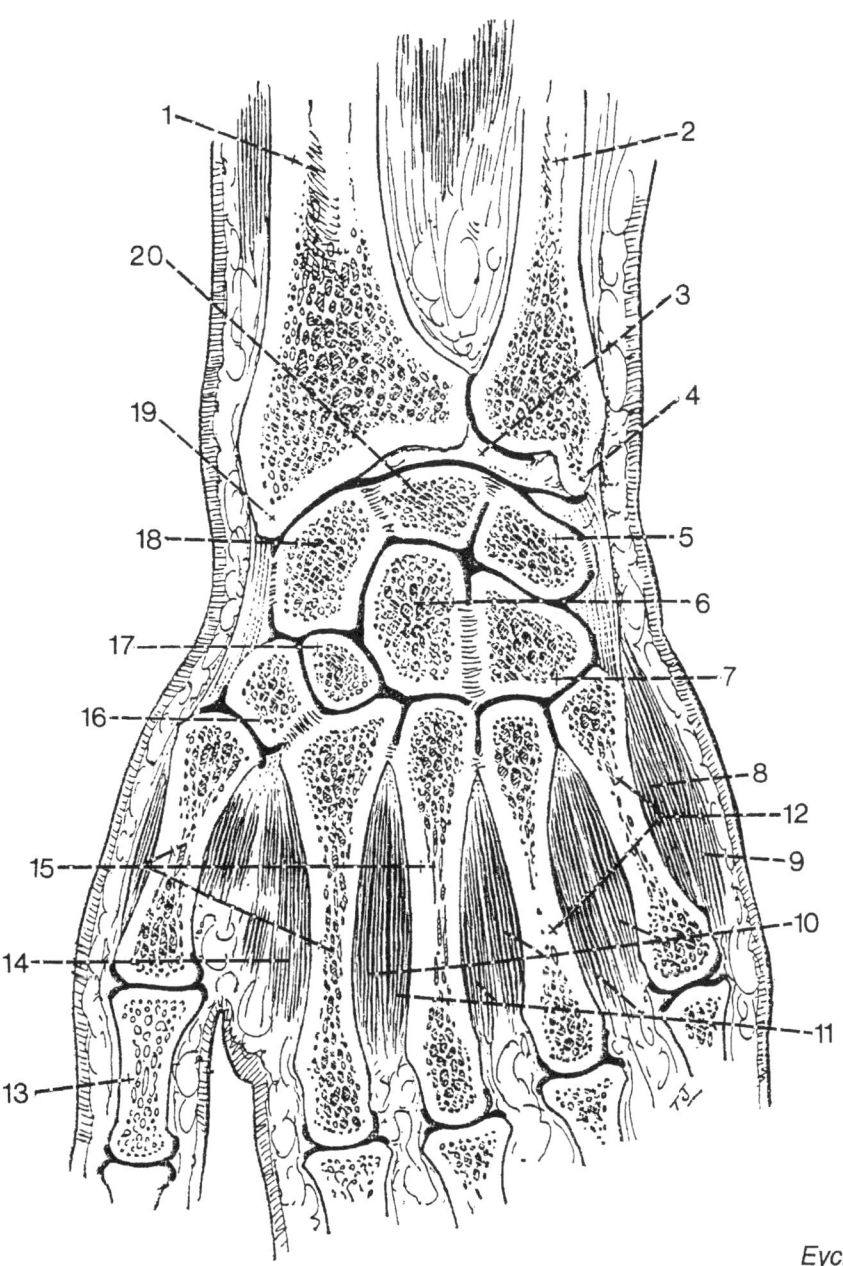

Eycleshymer and Jones

Color and label

1. Radius
2. Ulna
3. Articular disk
4. Styloid process of ulna
5. Triquetral bone (plane of section does not pass through pisiform)
6. Capitate bone
7. Hamate bone
8. Opponens digiti muscle
9. Abductor digiti minimi muscle
10. Palmar interosseous muscles
11. Dorsal interosseous muscles
12. Fourth and fifth metacarpal bones
13. Proximal phalanx of thumb
14. First dorsal interosseous muscle
15. First, second, and third metacarpal bones
16. Trapezium bone (old name, greater multangular)
17. Trapezoid bone (old name, lesser multangular)
18. Scaphoid bone (old name, navicular)
19. Styloid process of radius
20. Lunate bone

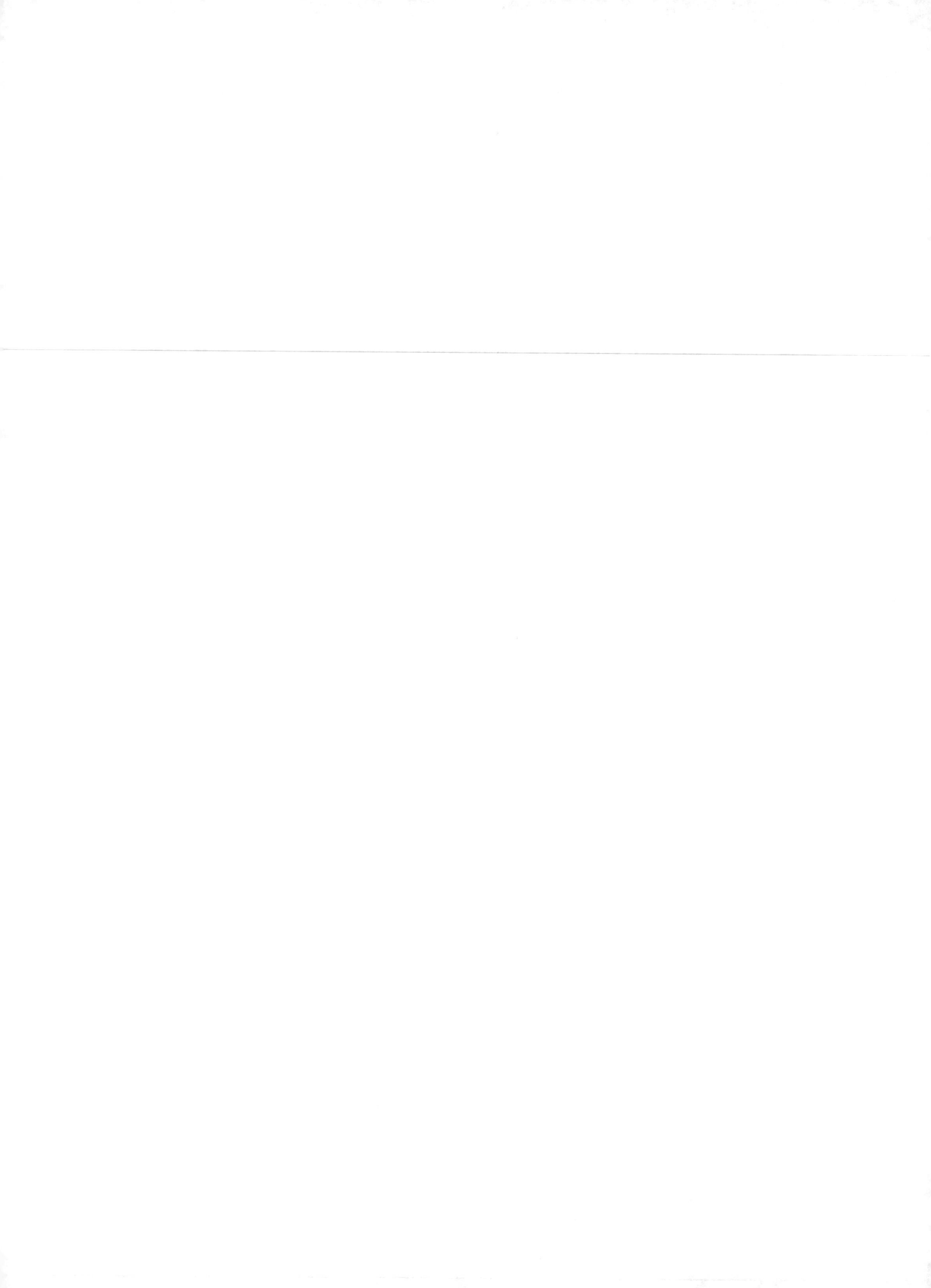

64 Coronal section of the right shoulder

(The glenoid cavity lies posterior to the plane of section)

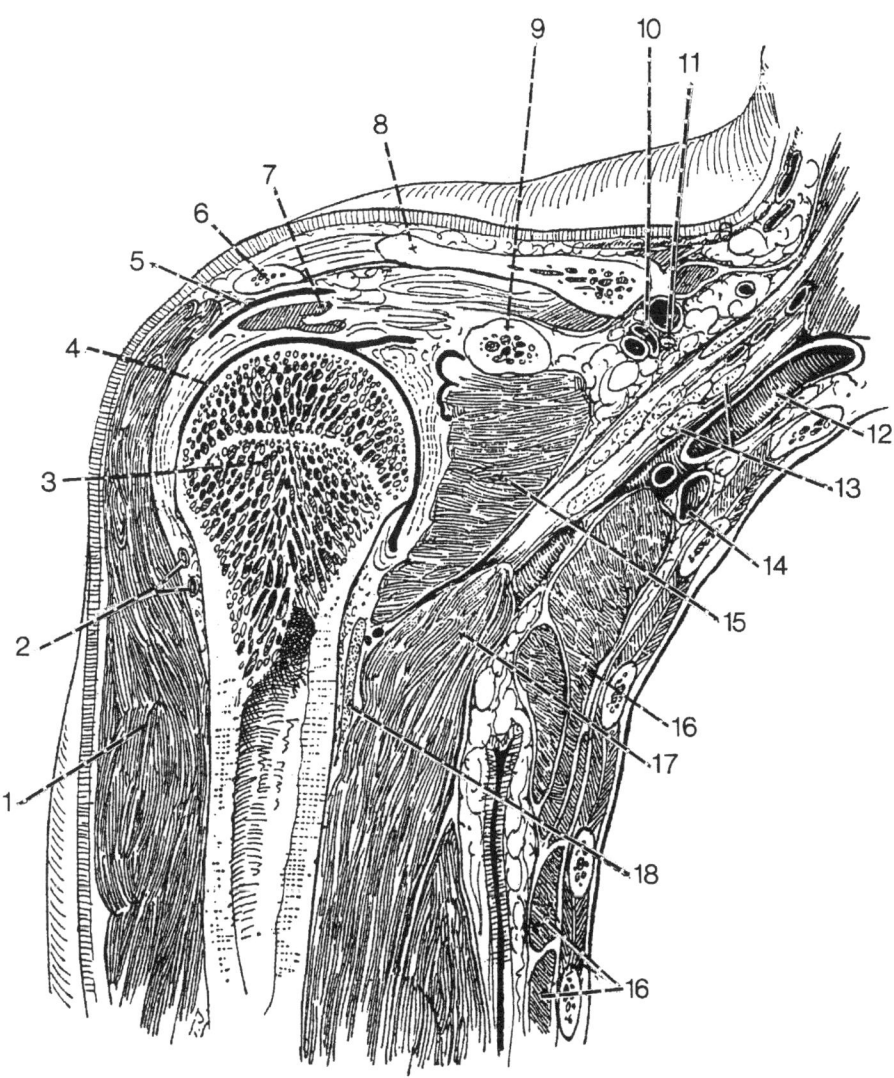

Eycleshymer and Jones

Color and label

1. Deltoid muscle
2. Posterior circumflex humeral artery and vein
3. Head of humerus
4. Articular cavity
5. Bursa
6. Acromion
7. Supraspinatus muscle
8. Clavicle
9. Coracoid process
10. Transverse scapular artery
11. Suprascapular nerve
12. Subclavian artery
13. Brachial plexus
14. Subclavian vein
15. Subscapular muscle
16. Serratus anterior muscle
17. Triceps brachii muscle (long head)
18. Tendon of latissimus dorsi

65 Ligaments of right shoulder joint

Anterior aspect

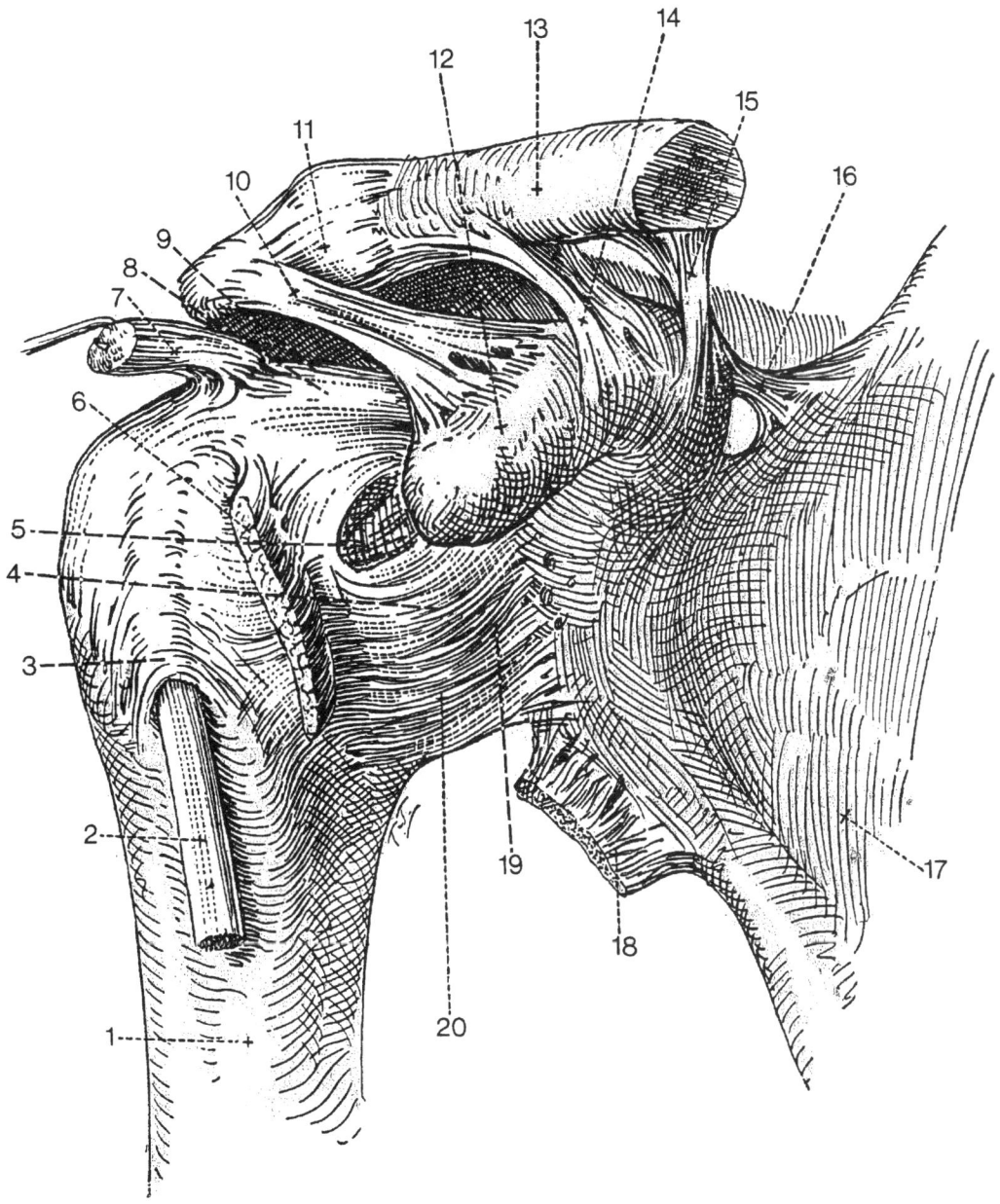

Eycleshymer and Jones

Color and label

1. Humerus
2. Biceps brachii (long head, tendon, cut)
3. Transverse humeral ligament
4. Middle glenohumeral ligament
5. Opening of subscapular bursa
6. Subscapularis muscle
7. Supraspinatus muscle (tendon, cut and pulled laterally)
8. Superior glenohumeral ligament
9. Coracohumeral ligament
10. Coracoacromial ligament
11. Acromioclavicular ligament
12. Coracoid process
13. Clavicle
14. Trapezoid ligament
15. Conoid ligament
16. Superior transverse scapular ligament
17. Scapula
18. Triceps brachii (long head)
19. Inferior glenohumeral ligament
20. Fibrous capsule of shoulder joint

66 Ligaments of right shoulder joint

Posterior aspect

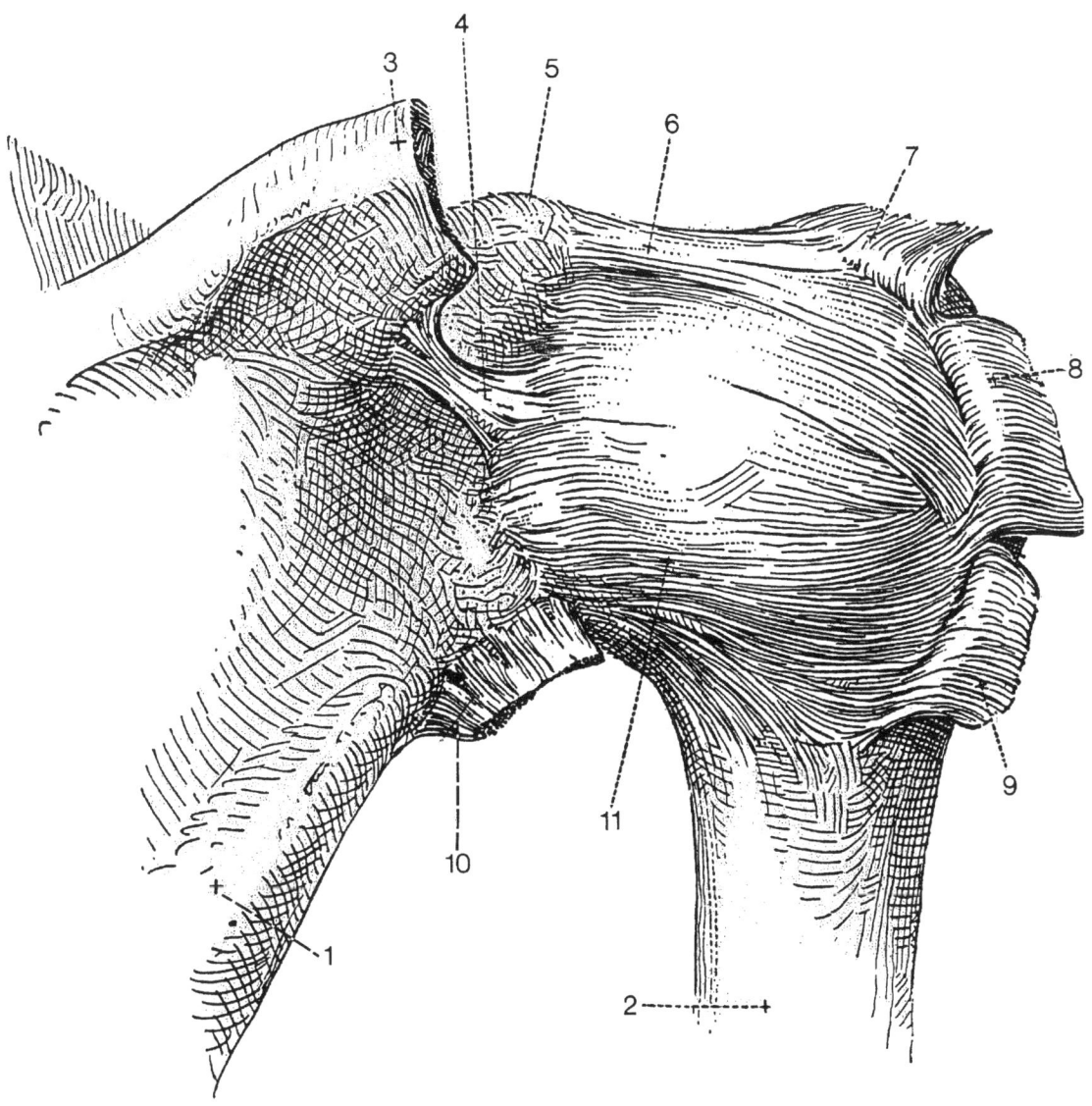

Eycleshymer and Jones

Color and label

1. Scapula (lateral part)
2. Humerus
3. Spine of scapula (acromion has been cut off)
4. Inferior transverse scapular ligament
5. Coracoid process
6. Coracohumeral ligament
7. Supraspinatus muscle (reflected and cut)*
8. Infraspinatus muscle (reflected and cut)*
9. Teres minor muscle (reflected and cut)*
10. Long head of triceps brachii (cut)
11. Articular capsule

*These three muscles plus the **subscapularis** make up the **rotator cuff.**

67 Ligaments of right elbow

Viewed from the ulnar side

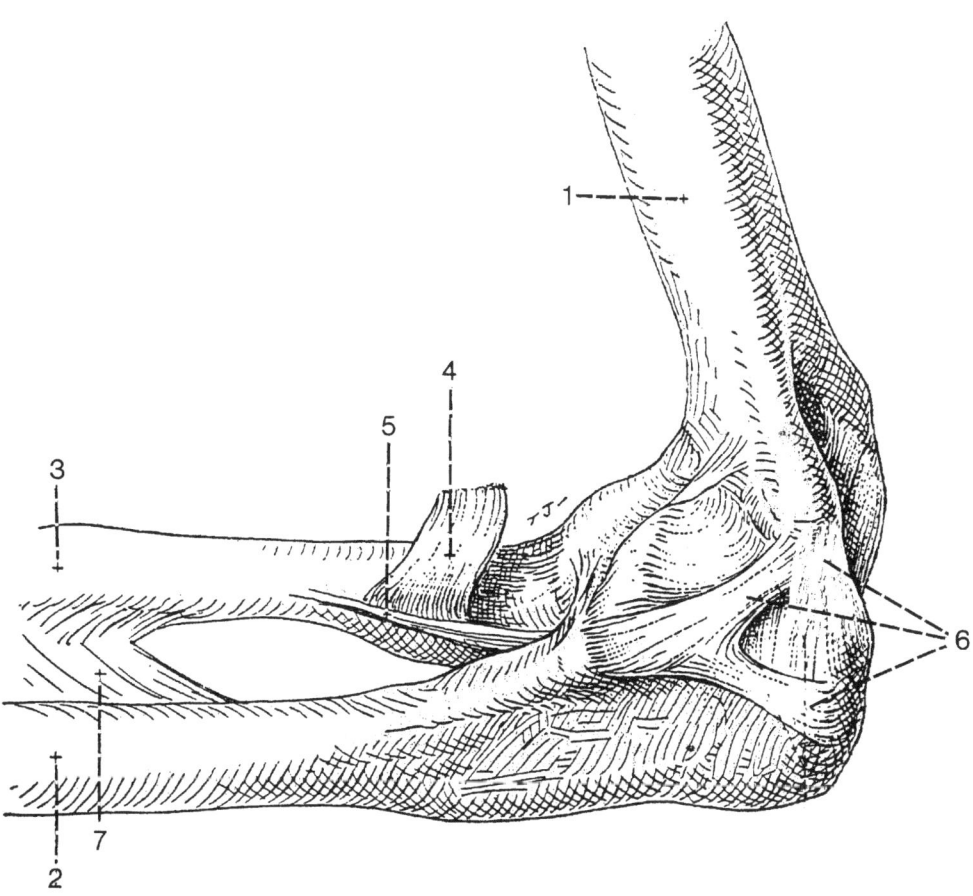

Color and label

1. Humerus
2. Ulna
3. Radius (forearm is supinated, radius and ulna are parallel, not crossed)
4. Tendon of biceps brachii inserting on radial tuberosity
5. Oblique cord
6. Ulnar collateral ligament
7. Interosseous membrane

Eycleshymer and Jones

68 Ligaments of right elbow

Anterior aspect

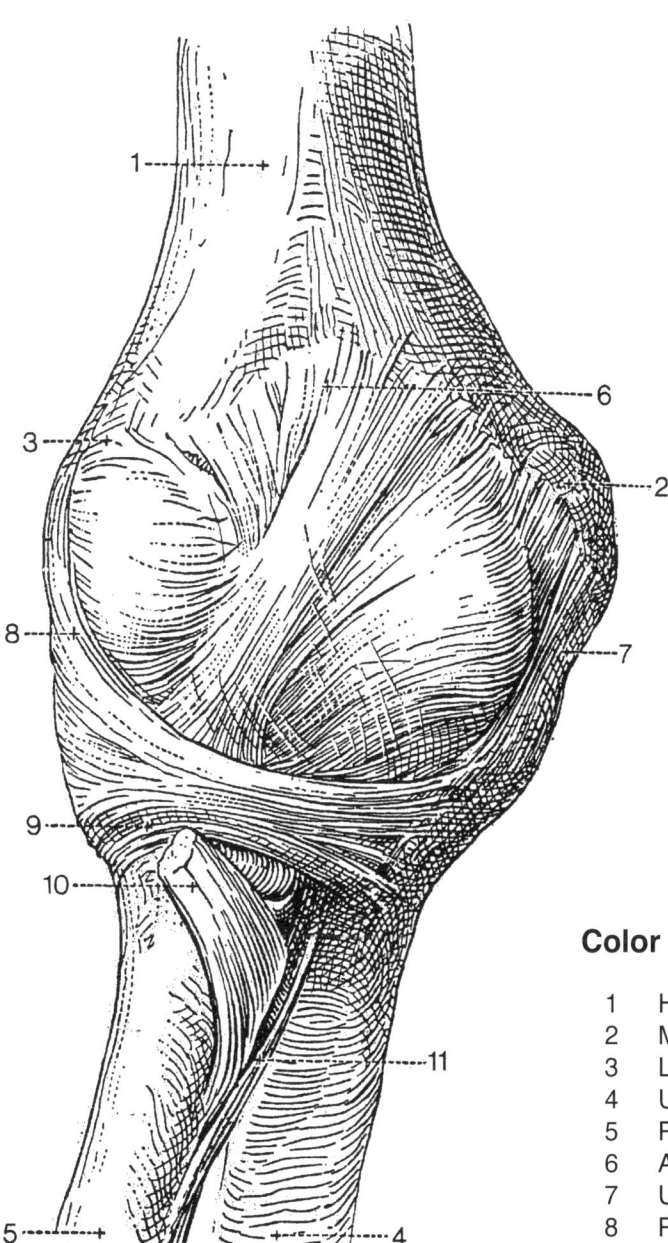

Eycleshymer and Jones

Color and label

1 Humerus
2 Medial epicondyle
3 Lateral epicondyle
4 Ulna
5 Radius
6 Articular capsule
7 Ulnar collateral ligament
8 Radial collateral ligament
9 Annular ligament of radius (surrounds head of radius) allows radius to rotate (supinate and pronate) on its longitudinal axis
10 Tendon of biceps brachii
11 Oblique cord

69 Sagittal section of right elbow

Viewed from the radial side

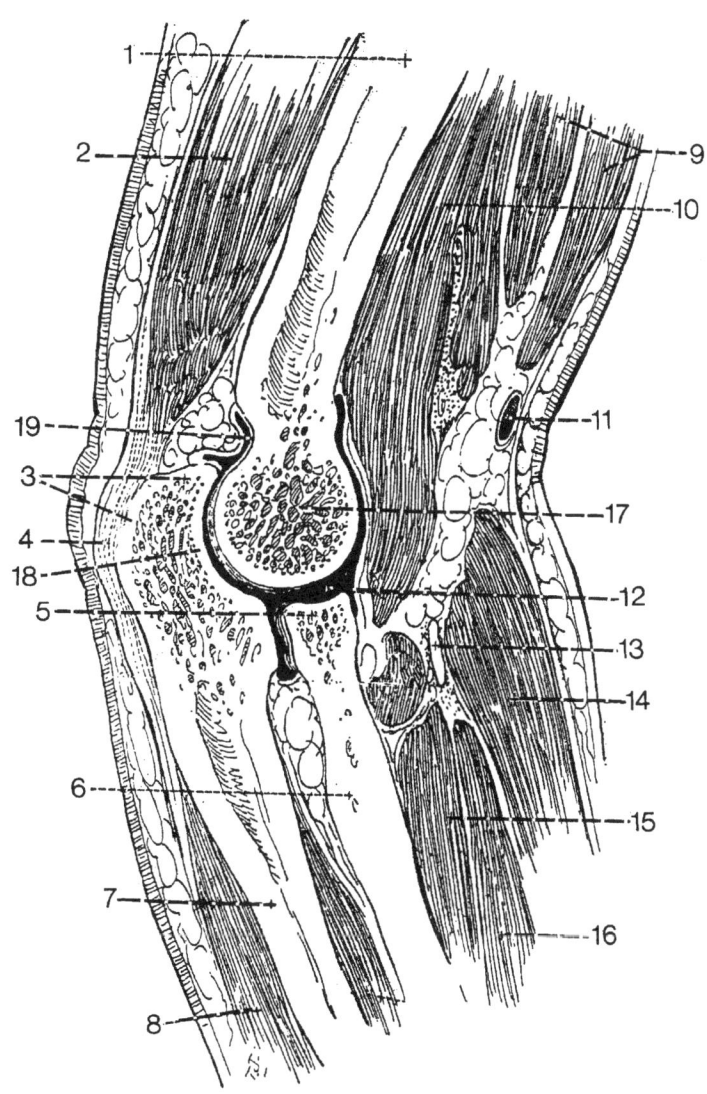

Color and label

1 Humerus
2 Triceps brachii muscle
3 Olecranon of ulna
4 Tendon of triceps brachii insertion on olecranon
5 Head of radius
6 Radius
7 Ulna
8 Flexor digitorum profundus muscle
9 Biceps brachii muscle
10 Brachialis muscle
11 Cephalic vein
12 Joint cavity
13 Radial nerve
14 Brachioradialis muscle
15 Supinator muscle
16 Extensor carpi radialis brevis muscle
17 Trochlea of humerus
18 Trochlear notch of ulna
19 Olecranon fossa of humerus

Eycleshymer and Jones

70 Frontal section of right elbow

Viewed from the front

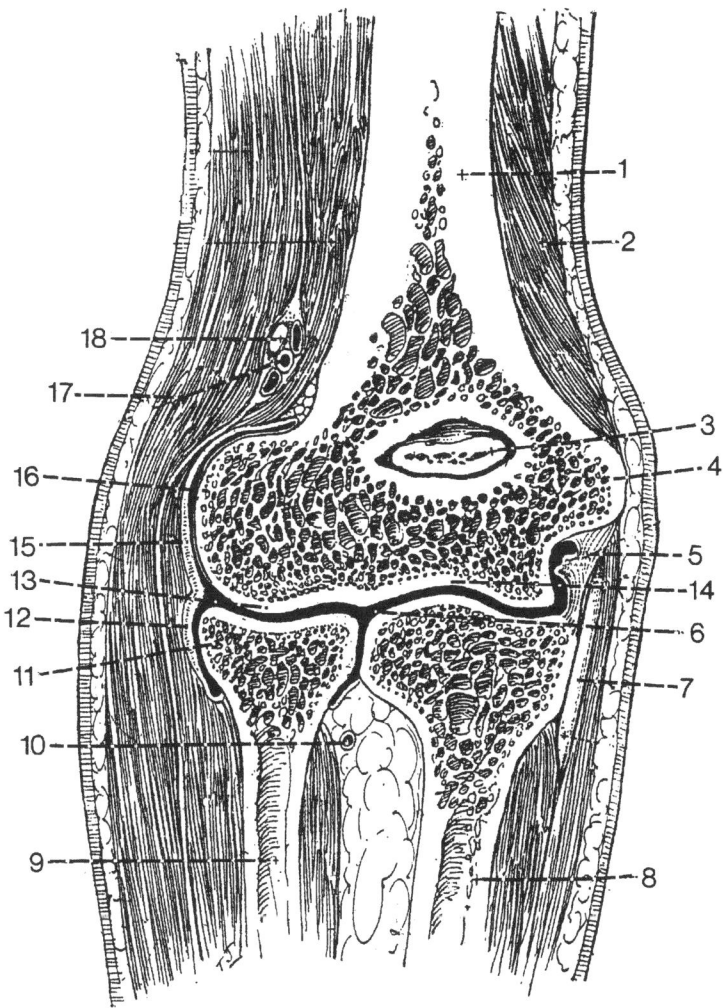

Elbow is extended so that olecranon lies in olecranon fossa of humerus

Color and label

1. Humerus
2. Brachialis muscle
3. Olecranon of ulna (in olecranon fossa of humerus)
4. Medial epicondyle of humerus
5. Articular capsule (internal to ulnar collateral ligament)
6. Articular cavity (joint cavity)
7. Ulnar nerve
8. Ulna
9. Radius
10. Common interosseous artery (branch of ulnar artery)
11. Head of radius
12. Annular ligament of radius
13. Capitulum of humerus
14. Trochlea of humerus
15. Radial collateral ligament
16. Lateral epicondyle of humerus
17. Radial collateral artery (branch of deep brachial artery) and accompanying veins
18. Radial nerve

Eycleshymer and Jones with modification

71 Ligaments of right wrist

Palmar aspect

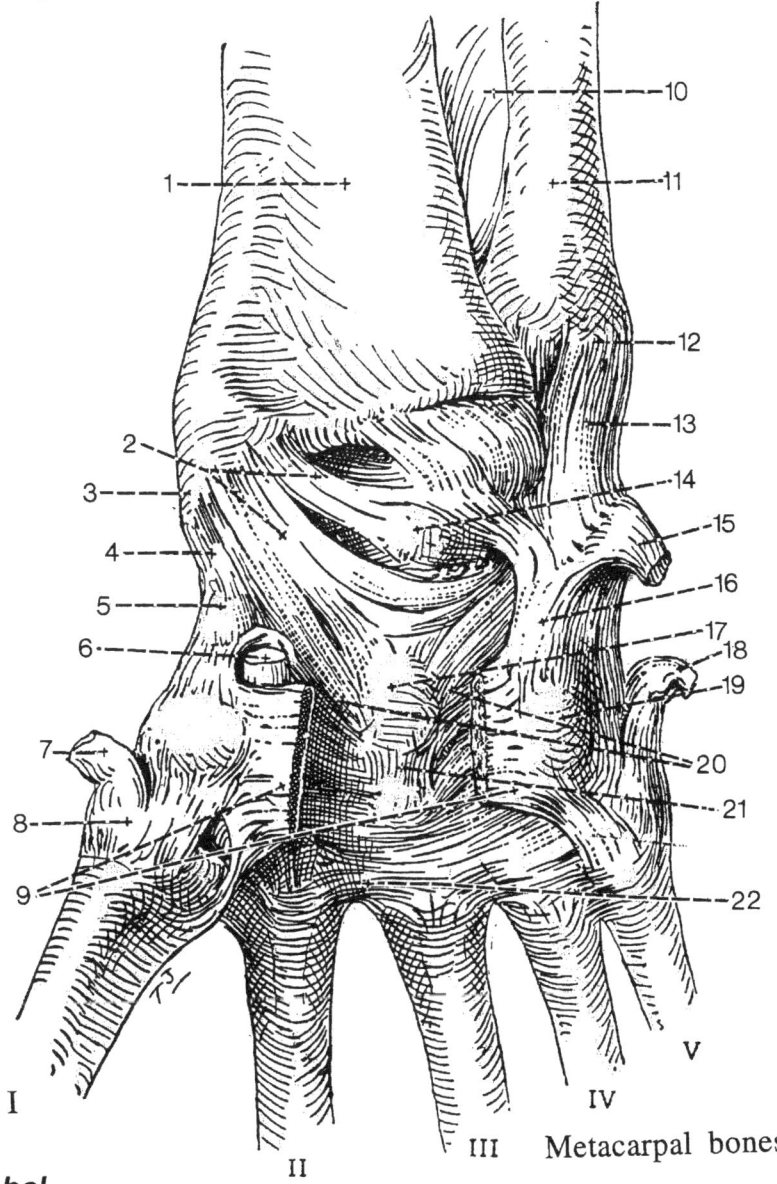

Color and label

1. Radius
2. Palmar radiocarpal ligament
3. Styloid process of radius
4. Radial collateral carpal ligament
5. Tubercle of trapezoid bone
6. Tendon of flexor carpi radialis insertion onto base of second metacarpal
7. Tendon of abductor pollicis longus insertion onto lateral side of base of first metacarpal and trapezium
8. Carpometacarpal joint of thumb
9. Flexor retinaculum (cut) (old name, transverse carpal ligament)
10. Interosseous membrane
11. Ulna
12. Styloid process of ulna
13. Ulnar carpal collateral ligament
14. Lunate bone
15. Tendon of flexor carpi ulnaris (cut) insertion onto the pisiform and by the pisohamate ligament and pisometacarpal ligament to the hamate bone and the base of the fifth metacarpal, respectively
16. Pisohamate ligament
17. Capitate bone
18. Tendon of extensor carpi ulnaris insertion on medial side of base of fifth metacarpal
19. Hamulus of hamate bone
20. Carpal radiating ligament
21. Palmar carpometacarpal ligament
22. Palmar (inter) metacarpal ligaments

Eycleshymer and Jones with modification

72 Ligaments of right wrist

Posterior aspect

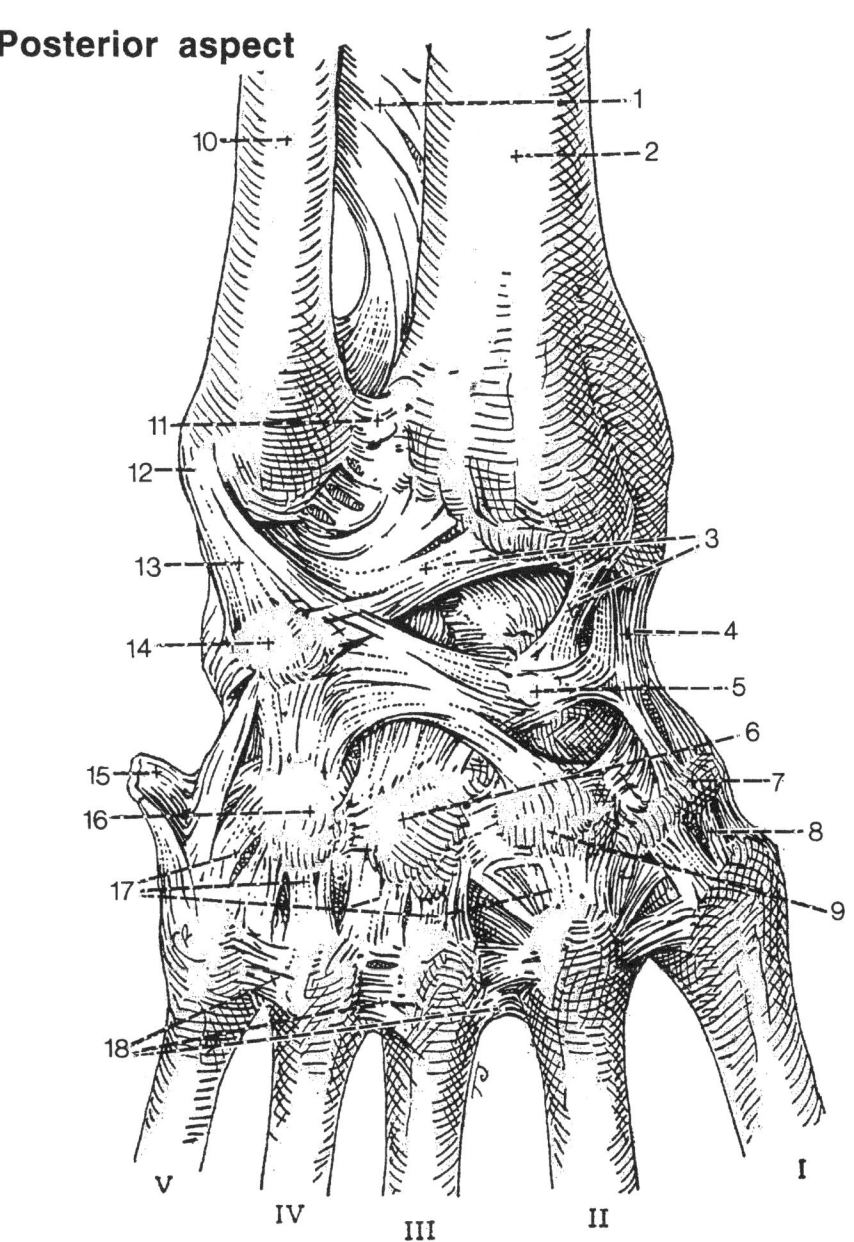

Metacarpal bones

Color and label

1. Antebrachial (forearm) interosseous membrane
2. Radius
3. Dorsal radiocarpal ligament
4. Radial carpal collateral ligament
5. Scaphoid bone (old name, navicular)
6. Capitate bone
7. Trapezium bone (old name, greater multangular)
8. Carpometacarpal joint of thumb (pollicis)
9. Trapezoid bone (old name, lesser multangular)
10. Ulna
11. Distal radial-ulnar joint (articulation)
12. Styloid process of ulna
13. Ulnar carpal collateral ligament
14. Triquetral bone
15. Tendon (cut) of extensor carpi ulnaris (insertion on base of fifth metacarpal)
16. Hamate bone
17. Dorsal carpometacarpal ligaments
18. Dorsal (inter) metacarpal (bases) ligaments

Eycleshymer and Jones

73 Hand dissection

Oblique view, palmar aspect
Skin and palmar aponeurosis removed

Oblique view Palmar aspect
Skin and palmar aponeurosis removed

Color and label

1. Tendon of flexor pollicis longus muscle
2. Adductor pollicis muscle muscle
3. First lumbrical muscle
4. Abductor pollicis brevis muscle
5. Radial artery
6. Cut end of tendon of palmaris longus
7. Ulnar artery
8. Ulnar nerve
9. Flexor retinaculum
10. Communicating branch of ulnar nerve with median nerve
11. Hypothenar muscles
12. Common palmar digital branches of median nerve

Figure 74
Figure 75
Figure 76

13. Superficial palmar (arterial) arch
14. Common palmar digital nerve and artery
15. Tendon of flexor digitorum superficialis muscle to 3rd finger
16. Tendon of flexor digitorum profundus
17. Proper palmar digital artery
18. Annular fibers of fibrous tendon sheath
19. Proper palmar digital nerve
20. Cruciate fibers of fibrous tendon sheath
21. Tendon of flexor digitorum superficialis muscle

74 Wrist cross-section

Right hand, looking up from below

Color and label

1. Flexor retinaculum; this forms the "roof" or ventral wall of the carpal tunnel
2. Ulnar artery
3. Ulnar nerve
4. Four tendons of flexor digitorum superficialis muscle
5. Hypothenar muscles
6. Hook (uncus) of hamate bone
7. Four tendons of flexor digitorum profundus muscle
8. Tendon of extensor carpi ulnaris muscle
9. Tendon of extensor digiti minimi muscle
10. Hamate bone (carpal bone)
11. Tendons of extensor digitorum muscle
12. Capitate bone (carpal bone)
13. Tendon of extensor indicis
14. Tendon of extensor carpi radialis brevis
15. Trapezoid bone (carpal bone)
16. Tendon of extensor carpi radialis longus muscle
17. Tendon of extensor pollicis longus muscle
18. Radial artery (in snuff box)
19. Cephalic vein
20. Trapezium (carpal bone)
21. Tendon of extensor pollicis brevis muscle
22. Tendon of abductor pollicis longus muscle
23. Opponens pollicis muscle
24. Tendon of flexor carpi radialis muscle
25. Tendon of flexor pollicis longus muscle
26. Abductor pollicis brevis muscle
27. Median nerve
28. Flexor pollicis brevis muscle
29. "Snuff box"

Ventral

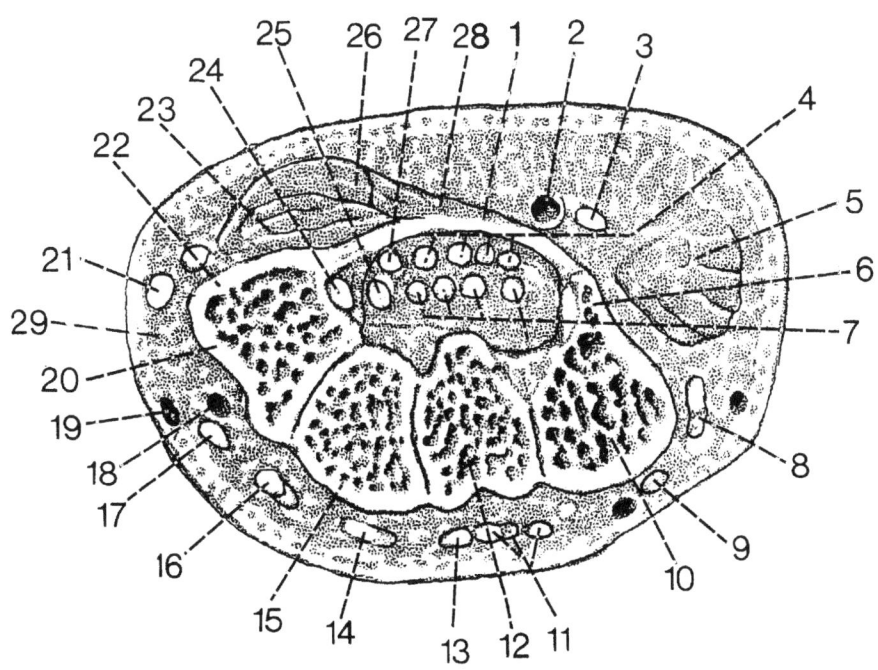

75 Hand cross-section I
Level of thumb metacarpal bone

Looking up from below

Color and label

1. First metacarpal bone (of thumb)
2. Opponens pollicis muscle
3. Abductor pollicis brevis muscle
4. Tendon of flexor pollicis longus muscle
5. Flexor pollicis brevis muscle
6. Median nerve and first lumbrical muscle
7. Tendons of flexor digitorum superficialis and flexor digitorum profundus to index finger
8. Palmar aponeurosis
9. Ulnar nerve and arterial branch off superficial palmar arch
10. Superficial and deep flexor tendons to fifth finger
11. Flexor digiti minimi muscle
12. Abductor digiti minimi muscle
13. Opponens digiti minimi muscle
14. Ventral (palmar or volar) interosseous muscle
15. Fifth metacarpal bone
16. Fourth dorsal interosseous muscle
17. Tendons of superficial flexor muscle and deep (profundus) flexor muscle to fourth finger (deep tendon is surrounded by third lumbrical muscle)
18. Fourth metacarpal bone bone
19. Third dorsal interosseous muscle
20. Tendons of superficial and deep flexor muscles to third finger (deep tendon is surrounded by second lumbrical muscle)
21. Third metacarpal bone
22. Second dorsal interosseous muscle
23. First ventral (palmar or volar) interosseous muscle
24. Second metacarpal bone
25. First dorsal interosseous muscle
26. Adductor pollicis muscle
27. Cephalic vein
28. Radial artery
29. Tendon of extensor pollicic brevis
30. Tendon of extensor pollicis longus
31. Tendon of extensor digitorum to 4th digit

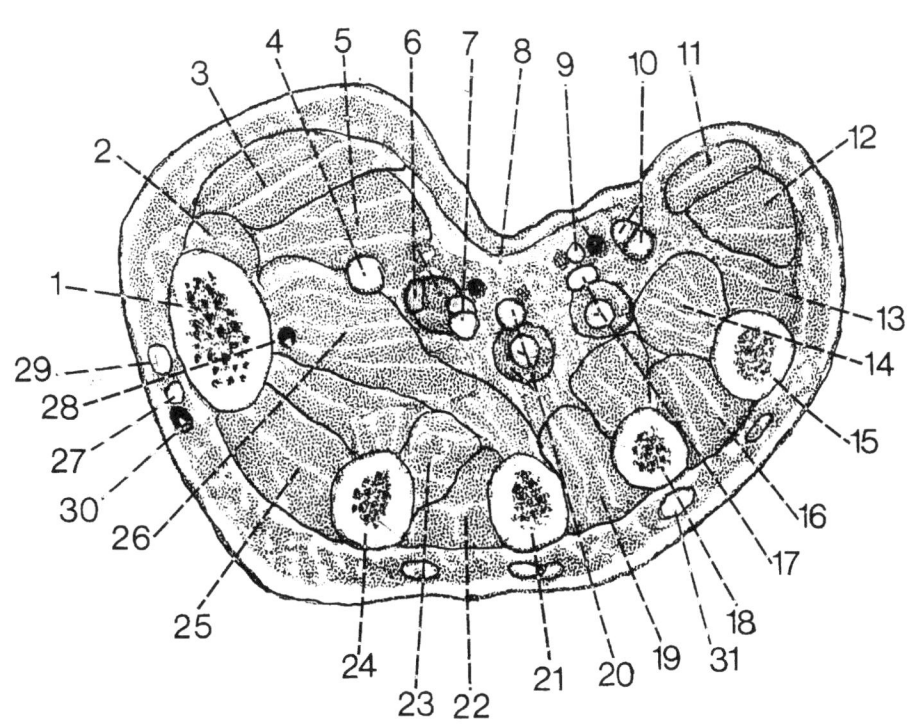

Ventral

76 Hand cross-section II

Heads of metacarpal bones 2-5

Looking up from below

Color and label

1. Tendon of extensor pollicis longus muscle
2. Distal phalanx of thumb
3. Tendon of flexor pollicis longus muscle
4. Superficial flexor tendons to digits 2-5
5. Deep flexor tendons to digits 2-5
6. Tendon of extensor digiti minimi
7. Extensor digitorum tendon to fifth finger
8. Fifth metacarpal
9. Extensor digitorum tendon to fourth finger
10. Fourth metacarpal bone
11. Extensor digitorum tendon to third finger
12. Extensor indicis tendon to second finger
13. Third metacarpal
14. Extensor digitorum tendon to second (index) finger
15. Second metacarpal
16. First lumbrical muscle
17. First dorsal interosseous muscle
18. Compartments for interosseous muscles
19. Neurovascular bundles to each finger

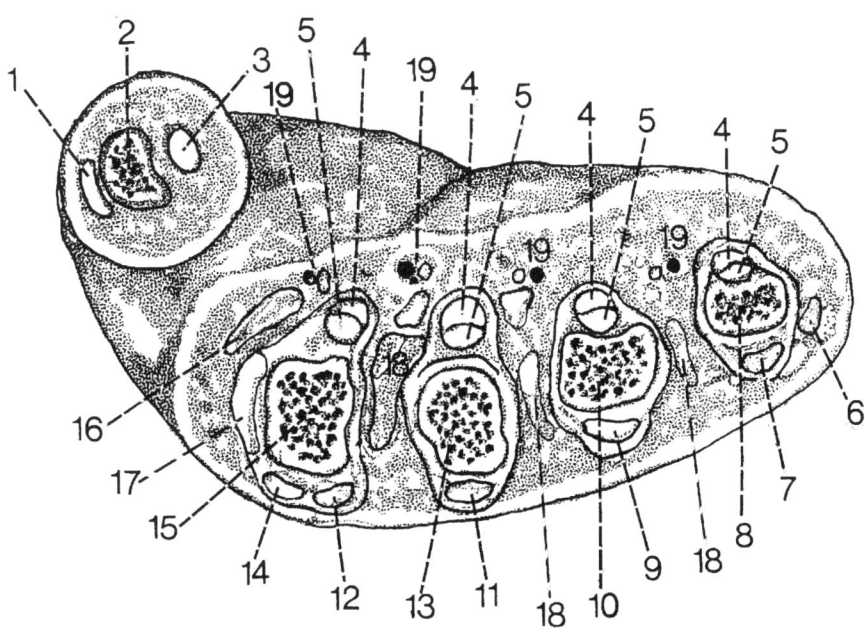

Ventral

77 Unlabelled bones of the hand for self study
Ventral aspect

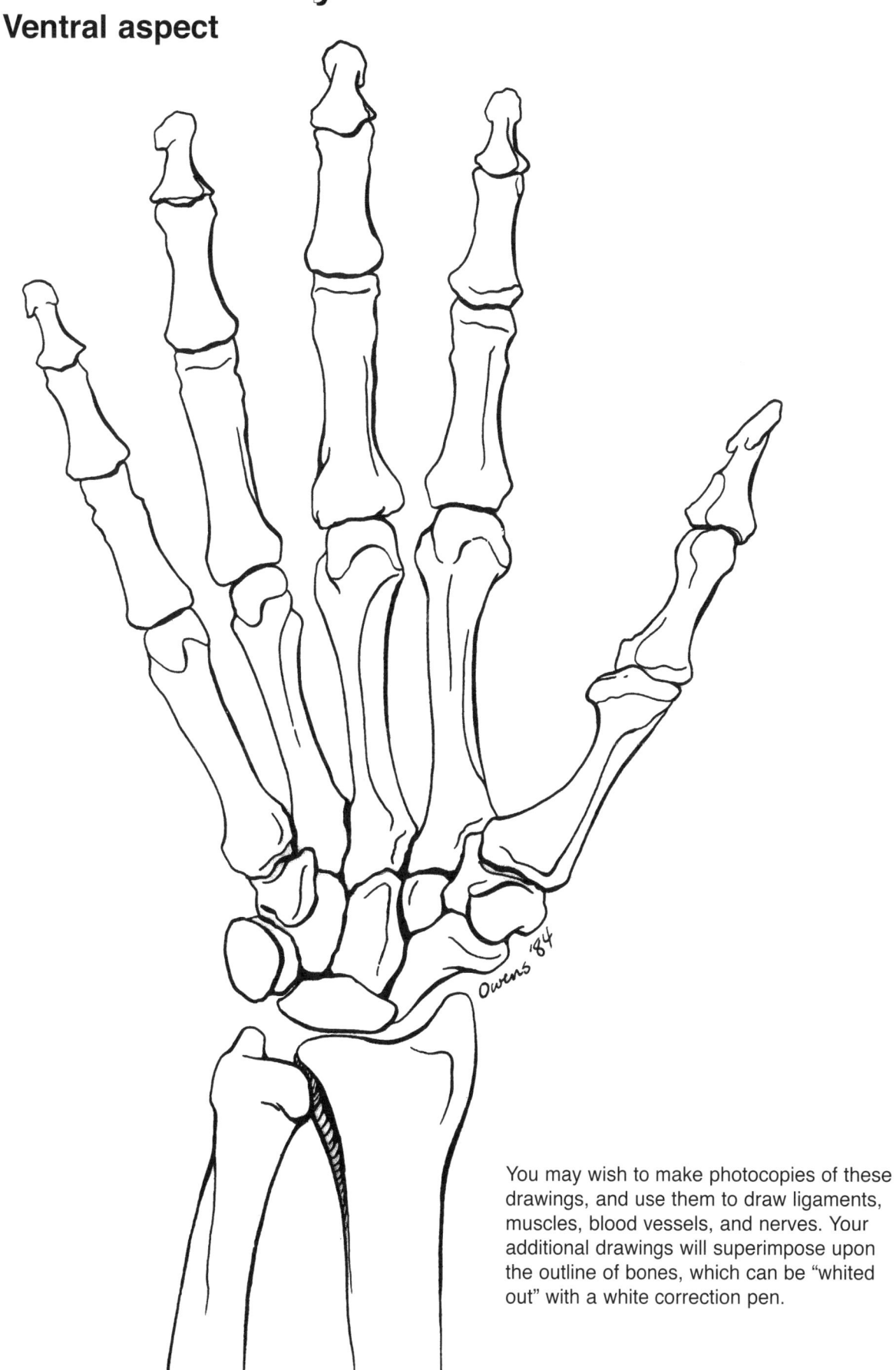

You may wish to make photocopies of these drawings, and use them to draw ligaments, muscles, blood vessels, and nerves. Your additional drawings will superimpose upon the outline of bones, which can be "whited out" with a white correction pen.

78 Unlabelled bones of the hand for self study
Dorsal aspect

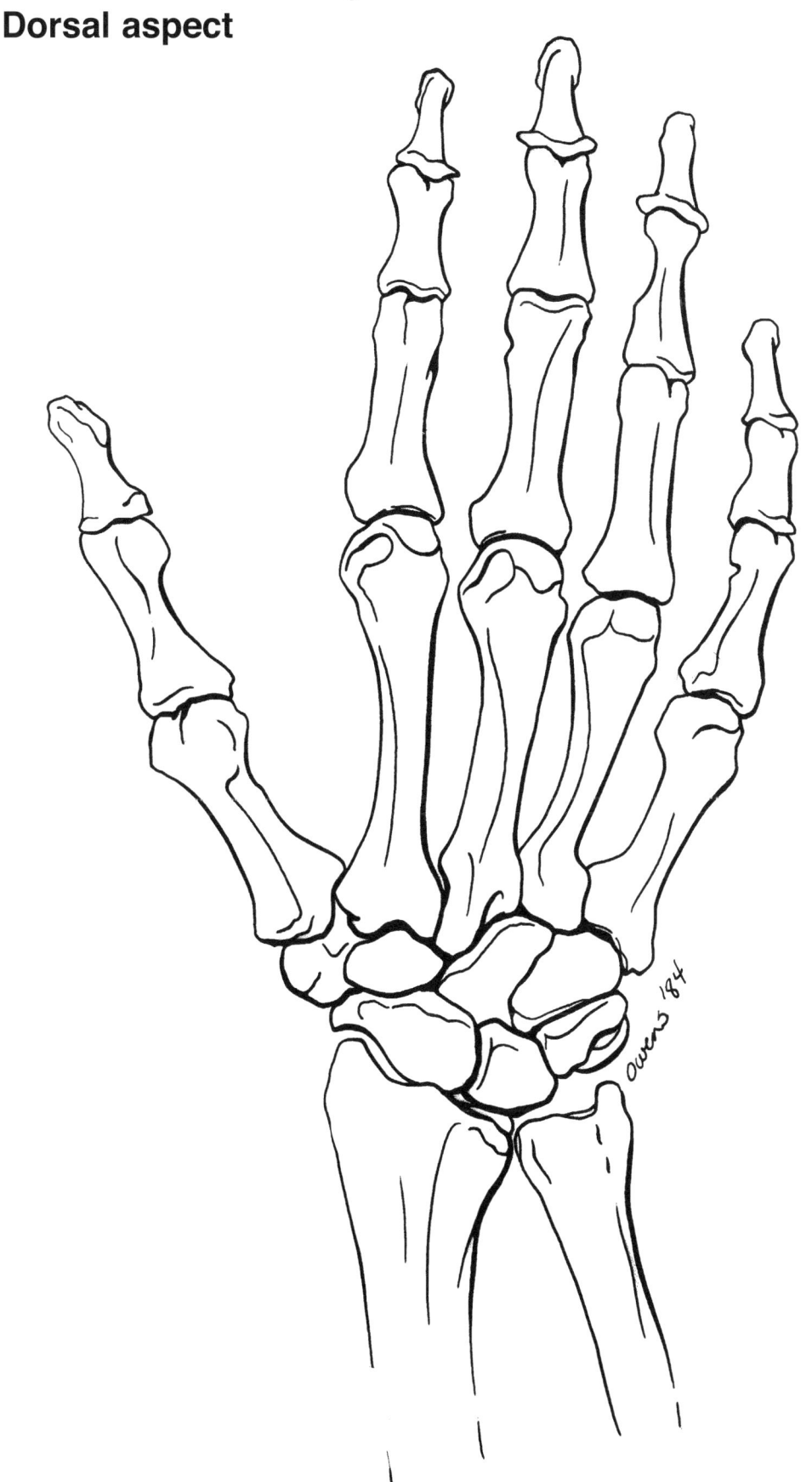